WOMEN'S WISDOM

NATURAL WELLNESS STRATEGIES FOR PREGNANCY

LAUREL ALEXANDER

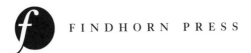

FINDHORN PRESS

The right of Laurel Alexander to be identified as the author
of this work has been asserted by her in accordance
with the Copyright, Designs and Patents Act 1998.

Published in 2012 by Findhorn Press, Scotland

ISBN 978-1-84409-585-8

A CIP record for this title is available from the British Library.

Edited by Nicky Leach
Cover design and illustrations by Richard Crookes
Yoga picture on cover © Ryan Libre, Documentary Arts Asia
Interior design by Damian Keenan
Printed and bound in the EU

1 2 3 4 5 6 7 8 9 17 16 15 14 13 12

Published by
Findhorn Press
117-121 High Street,
Forres IV36 1AB,
Scotland, UK

t +44 (0)1309 690582
f +44 (0)131 777 2711
e info@findhornpress.com
www.findhornpress.com

CONTENTS

Introduction

My journey towards writing this book began more than 10 years ago. As a complementary therapist and wellness coach, I began to notice the increase in the amount of pregnant women coming to me. It was not because I advertised, because nearly all my business comes from word of mouth. Still, women would contact me saying they wanted to conceive; they wanted reflexology as part of their natural pregnancy care; they were suffering from sickness, digestive problems, or some other pregnancy symptom; they were near their birthing time and they wanted a natural birth. Would I help them?

I am a complementary therapist – tick that box. I am a woman – I can tick that one, too. But I am not a mother. How can I help these women who come to me when I haven't been a mother myself? I eventually learnt to trust that these women seemed to instinctively know I was right for them.

Now, 10 years later, I understand how privileged I am to be able to walk with women on their journey of conception, pregnancy, and post-natal care. I have worked with women who have gone through multiple miscarriages and gone on to successfully conceive and give birth. I have worked with women going through IVF who have become pregnant, and with women who have tragically lost their babies at only months old and who have had the courage to conceive and give birth again. I have worked with first-time mums, helping them through their anxieties, and with second- and third-time mums celebrating further additions to their family.

Why haven't I had children of my own when so much of my work is with women and birthing? The timing and the circumstances never seemed right. Then when I was diagnosed with breast cancer at 39 (I'm 53 at the time of writing this book) and had to spend the next five years on tamoxifen, the opportunity seemed finally closed. It was a sad time for my husband and I when we understood this, but now my mothering instincts find expression with my life partner, with clients and students, with my friends, and with the animals with whom I share my life.

My interest in the philosophy of the Wise Woman Tradition spans many years. For me, the weave of ancient eclectic beliefs and values combined with practical application and modern psychology has provided a natural pathway for understanding the milestones in my life. In this book, I would like to share with you some of the tools I use with pregnant women and which you may like to work with on your special journey through your pregnancy. Choose instinctively, and travel with Spirit.

— Laurel

A Wysecraft Tale
for Pregnancy

The Pillar of Light moves across space and time as a flash of gold seen from the corner of your eye. It travels across the lush and undulating hills that cover the summer landscape—skims the gentle wind that whispers through the grasses and slips over the gentle slopes and long vistas of the land. It dances through the clear morning sun and moves lazily into the shimmering afternoon, before sliding into the duskiness of evening and blending into the dark mystery of night.

The Pillar of Light listens to the song of summer animals, breathes in the fragrance of flowers, and celebrates the richness, fertility, warmth, and colour of the high season. The Pillar of Light feels the joy of nature. High summer is the season of expansion and of reaching out into life. Anything is possible.

The Pillar of Light travels across the earth as the land flexes and stretches its shape languidly beneath the heat of the sun. The light and warmth reflects the self-confidence of female fertility as they move through the undulating sweep of groves and hills. Balmy nights wrap a rippling swath of grey-and-black chiffon over the curvaceous land and hint at ripe sexuality and hidden folds.

The summer rains, fine mist, and morning dew moisten the land deep into the crevices and ripen the dark richness for impregnation of new growth. The fertile earth is as a woman's womb. There is a sense of leisurely lustiness as the land spreads herself open. Soft and yielding.

The Pillar of Light travels farther along the valley with a hill on either side. It moves among the curves and crevices towards a hidden entrance, protected by the most perfumed of flowering bushes. The Pillar of Light symbolizes the Sun God and his glory. The summer cauldron of the land represents the sacredness of the Earth Goddess and her lush bounty.

A wondrous sunrise greets the dawn, as the Pillar of Light pierces the east-facing hill and the opening to the most sacred of female places. The wetness of the earth softens to receive the Pillar of Light, co-creating a divine spark of life in its symbolism of the universal womb. As the two energies entwine deep within the earth, an intense focal point of incredible energy builds. All the land is aroused from deep within as the creative force seeks expression. Rhythmic surges engulf the land in ecstatic release, and a glimpse of infinity infuses everything.

On this day of conception, as summer reaches its zenith overhead, the veil between this world and the fairy world of magick is stretched thinnest. The Summer Solstice is the longest day of the year. The God in his aspect as the Sun King is at his most powerful and at his side rules the Goddess as the Summer Queen, whose cauldron is filled with the bounty of the season of growth: ripe fruit and golden grain. As the sun descends into the power of the night, the moon rises to shed slivers of silver light on that which cloaks the new source of life.

In the darkest of places, deep down within the core of the earth, is a dark cave. The gateway of the cave is small and tight. The cave itself curves around, above, and beneath an embryo, which contains the beginnings of a brain, spinal cord, and heart, with the merest hint of arms and legs.

Time passes. Major organs and external body structures have begun to form within what is now a fetus. Its heartbeat pulsates around the cave. A silver cord links the fetus to the cave and therefore to the land. Time passes. The tiny fetus begins to move and grow. Its closed eyelids protect the developing eyes. Time passes. Muscle tissue and bone continue to form, creating a more complete skeleton. Skin begins to form, although it is almost transparent. The fetus makes sucking motions with its mouth.

Time passes. Eyebrows, eyelashes, fingernails, and toenails have formed. The fetus can hear and swallow and becomes more active. The cave walls ripple in response to the movement, and the land moves in contentment. Gently, the fetus tumbles and floats in the moist air of the cave. Time passes. The fetus is beginning to explore the cave wall, cord, and its own body parts. It responds to sound and reacts to light and dark.

Bone marrow begins to make blood cells. Taste buds form on the tongue of the fetus. Footprints and fingerprints have formed. Real hair begins to grow on the head of the fetus. The lungs are forming and the hands develop. The fetus sleeps and wakes regularly. It stores fat, has gained weight, and is now much bigger.

Time passes. The bones of the fetus are now fully formed but still soft. Its eyes open and close in response to changes in light. It kicks and jabs. Its lungs are not fully formed, but slight breathing movements occur. The fetus is gaining weight quickly and is even bigger. Time passes. Within the cave, there is the pulsating sound of Earth Mother's life blood and the steady beating of the land's heart. Noises from far outside the cave are muffled. As the fetus becomes bigger it has more body fat and less space to move around.

Time passes. The fetus is now full term and its organs are ready to function on their own. There is a moment where time holds its breath in anticipation. Now is the moment. High in the sky, the full moon holds her belly ready to give birth. The silver light bathes the land in preparation.

The cave walls, floor, and ceiling begin to surge in a rhythmic pattern, guiding the fetus, head first, to the gateway of the cave. The waiting fetus pauses as the gateway begins to soften and open. The pool of crystal clear water just outside the gateway suddenly cascades down the tunnel outside the cave. A powerful surge ripples through the gateway, opening it to its fullest potential and the fetus begins its journey through the opening.

The fetus is slowly propelled down the tunnel by a continuing series of pulsations. The earth breathes a steady rhythm, which the fetus picks up and integrates into its journey.

The fetus pauses in a plateau of serenity, as it transits into a small cave with moist, smooth walls. The light is dim and the air hot and humid as the fetus moves through the sacred cave of Yoni. Placing its head down, the fetus wears the crown of birth as the opening to Yoni moves over its head and body.

Finally, the baby is born to the outside world. The fine, silver energy mist surrounding the baby shimmers and moves through the dense, powerful energy of Earth Mother until the two energies are as one.

The baby rests upon the breast of the land, immersed in and surrounded by unconditional love. Travelling in the wake of the baby is a pulsating mass that includes the umbilical cord. With a final surge, the mass is expelled and when the pulsations have ceased, the cord dissolves and the divine source of life closes quietly over the land. The baby lies upon the waiting mother, who creates a cradle of summer herbs and flowers for her baby made of chamomile, lavender, rosemary, marigold, and jasmine. The baby has grown within the mother—their journey of two joined in one. Their spirit and soul have woven together, their sacred energies blended from the Divine. Yet as two they must grow. Their journey will take them through terrains of forest, valley, and grove and many rivers and streams to be crossed. Sun, rain, wind, and fire will be encountered as darkness and light show the way. Their journey will be full of opportunity. Sometimes they will travel together and sometimes separately, but never losing the sacred bond of mother and child.

Now is the start of their journey into a lifetime.

CHAPTER 1

Moving Through Pregnancy

Pregnancy lasts around 40 weeks, from the first day of your last normal period. These weeks are grouped into three trimesters.

First Trimester (weeks 1–12)

Hormonal changes may include: headaches, fatigue, nausea, pregnancy sickness (I don't call it morning sickness as it can occur 24/7 for many women), cravings or distaste for certain foods, mood swings, constipation, needing to wee more often, heartburn, and tender, swollen breasts with darkening nipples and areolas.

The embryo produces the hormone human chorionic gonadotrophin, which is in your body for the first 12 weeks of your pregnancy; this is the hormone that makes your pregnancy test positive. Early on, other pregnancy hormones are produced by the ovaries, while the placenta produces hormones from 12 weeks onwards. These hormones influence the growth of the fetus, are responsible for changes in your body, and initiate birthing.

Baby's changes

At four weeks, the developing baby is an embryo, with the suggestion of a brain and spinal cord. The fifth week sees the start of the period where the embryo's heart, brain, and spinal cord begin to form. At this point the embryo is made up of three layers of different kinds of cells:

- **TOP:** This layer becomes the embryo's skin, central and peripheral nervous systems, inner ear, eyes, and connective tissue.

- **MIDDLE:** This layer becomes the heart and the beginning of the circulatory system, bones, muscles, and kidneys.
- **INNER:** This layer becomes the intestine, lungs, and bladder.

In the sixth and seventh week, the brain, basic facial features and arms and legs develop. At eight weeks and nearly one inch in length, the embryo starts moving. All the major organs and external body structures are taking shape. The arms and legs grow longer, and we can see the beginnings of fingers and toes. The sex organs begin to form. The eyes have moved forward on the face and eyelids have taken shape. The umbilical cord is visible. The embryo's heart beats with a regular rhythm.

At 12 weeks, the embryo is a fetus of around three inches. The nerves and muscles begin to work together, the fetus can make a fist and we can see if it is a girl or a boy. The eyelids close to protect the developing eyes and will not open again until around week 28.

> **WISE WOMAN WAYS**
> If you experience bleeding (bright red blood) or cramps during your pregnancy, see your doctor as you may be starting to miscarry. You are likely to be sent to the hospital for a scan to check all is well.

Second Trimester (weeks 13–28)

As your body changes to make room for the growing fetus, you may have:
- Body aches;
- Stretch marks on your breasts, abdomen, buttocks, or thighs;
- A line on the skin from belly button to pubic hairline;
- Patches of darker skin on the face
- Numb or tingling hands (carpal tunnel syndrome);

- Itching on the abdomen, palms, and soles of the feet (consult your doctor, midwife, or doula if you have nausea, loss of appetite, vomiting, jaundice, or fatigue combined with itching, as these may be signs of a liver problem);
- Swelling of the ankles, fingers, and face (consult your doctor midwife or doula if you notice any sudden or extreme swelling or if you gain a lot of weight quickly as this could be a sign of preeclampsia).

Baby's changes

When the fetus is 16 weeks and about five inches in length, muscle tissue and bone continue to form and transparent skin is created. Meconium, the fetus's first stool movement, develops in the fetal intestinal tract. The fetus makes sucking motions with its mouth.

At 20 weeks with a length of around six inches, the fetus develops lanugo, a downy hair, on its body. A waxy-white coating called vernix coats the skin of the fetus, protecting it from the surrounding amniotic fluid. Eyebrows, eyelashes, fingernails, and toenails have formed. The fetus can hear and swallow.

When the fetus is 24 weeks old and 12 inches long, bone marrow begins to make blood cells. Taste buds form on the tongue of the fetus. Foot and finger prints are present. Real hair begins to grow on the head of the fetus. The lungs are formed, but do not work. The fetus sleeps and wakes regularly. If the fetus is a girl, her ovaries and uterus will be in place. If he is a boy, his testicles begin to move down from the abdomen into the scrotum. The fetus stores fat and is gaining weight.

> **WISE WOMAN WAYS**
> It is during the second trimester, around the 20th week, that movement of the fetus, or the "quickening," can be felt.

Third Trimester (weeks 29–40)

New body changes you might notice include:

- Shortness of breath as baby gets bigger and puts pressure on your lungs;
- Heartburn;
- Swelling of ankles, fingers, and face (consult your doctor or midwife in case of sudden or extreme swelling, or if you gain a lot of weight quickly; could be sign of preeclampsia);
- Feeling the baby "roll," which might cause discomfort;
- Piles, or hemorrhoids;
- Tender breasts, which may leak a watery pre-milk called colostrum;
- Your belly button sticking out;
- Your belly dropping due to the fetus turning in a downward position ready for birth;
- Insomnia;
- Increased desire to wee, as the fetus puts extra pressure on your bladder;
- "Head engagement," or "baby drop," where the fetus's head descends into your pelvic cavity releasing pressure on your upper abdomen and easing your breathing;
- Surges, which can be a sign of real or false birthing.

As you near your due date, your cervix becomes thinner and softer (called effacing). This is a normal, natural process that helps the birth canal (vagina) to open during the birthing process.

Baby's changes

By 32 weeks, the fetus is around 15 inches in length. Its bones are soft but fully formed, making its kicks and jabs a tad forceful. The eyes of the fetus open and close and can sense light. Slight breathing movements occur as the lungs start to fill out. The body of the fetus begins to store minerals. Lanugo begins to fall off.

By 36 weeks, the fetus is around 17 inches long. The vernix is getting thicker. Body fat increases.

By the end of 37 weeks, the fetus is considered full term, with organs ready to function on their own. It now weighs six to nine pounds and is 19-21 inches long.

JANE'S JOURNEY

I started working with Laurel towards the end of my first IVF (in vitro fertilization) cycle, in September 2010. When this cycle was unsuccessful, Laurel helped me to explore and understand my feelings of grief, frustration, and despair and worked with me to help me to prepare for the next IVF cycle, both emotionally and practically. I used journaling to help me externalize my thoughts and feelings, as well as the Australian Bush Essences to help me deal with some of my turbulent emotions. With the fantastic news that the second IVF attempt had worked (February 2011), I continued to work with Laurel, as I found it really valuable to reflect on my changing perceptions and emotions about being pregnant and becoming a mother. Laurel helped me handle issues relating to morning sickness, disturbed sleep and my changing emotions.

What Happens Next?

As we can see, there are medically defined stages as we move through pregnancy. But when we look at pregnancy through female spirituality, we move away from the scientific way of understanding this time in a woman's life into the profoundly empowering realms that can help us celebrate the rites of passage to the Mother Goddess. Read on to discover your connection with the Mother Goddess.

CHAPTER 2

Celebrating the Mother Goddess

The word "goddess" means a female divine being. Around the world, for thousands of years, many societies have worshipped a divine and powerful Mother Goddess, and goddess images of great antiquity have been found, dating back to 35,000 years BC or earlier.

Hunter-Gatherer Societies

Until about 8,000 BC, our ancestors organized themselves into hunter-gatherer societies with primitive religious beliefs that revolved around their land-based lifestyle. Hunting was pivotal to tribal survival, and as a result, the hunter element in society (mostly men) tended to worship hunting gods and animals, such as the God of the Hunt or the Stag Horned God (or buffalo).

Women were mostly the gatherer element in society. They took care of the tribe and were the child bearers and healers. The female life-giving principle was considered divine, and the importance of fertility and birthing in crops, animals, and in the tribe itself was crucial to survival. As a result, women in hunter-gatherer societies tended to worship vegetative goddesses. While men and women might have worshipped similar gods and goddesses within the tribal community, they may also have gravitated to gender-specific worship. Women experienced a connection between their bodies and the phases of the moon that further enhanced the mystical link with the moon and the goddess deity. Because of these links, women during this time tended to lead the spiritual rituals of the tribe.

As society evolved, people began to settle in one place, growing food and breeding animals. This was when they became paganized (the word "pagan" is derived from the Latin word *paganus,* meaning "country dweller"). Paganism originates from the Neolithic (Stone Age) era. It was thought that everything had a spirit, so people had gods and goddesses for all aspects of their lives, including nature. Civilizations developed, and the gods were adapted to the changing lives of the people to play an important role in every aspect of the community.

The Triple Goddess

Long before the advent of Christianity, the Temple in Jerusalem had a tower representing the Great Goddess in her triple aspect. Known as Mari (a possible ancient Goddess source influencing the later worship of Mary and the Virgin Mother), the images shown are the three stages of the female life cycle: the premenstrual maiden, the fertile menstrual nymph, and the postmenopausal crone.

Neopagan is a broad definition used for a wide variety of modern religious or spiritual concepts influenced by the pre-Christian pagan beliefs of Europe. Wicca (popularly called White Witchcraft, the benign religion of the ancient Celts and an example of neopaganism) reemerged in the mid-20th century in England. Not only does Wicca tend to honour the Triple Goddess of Maiden (virginity), Mother (fertility), and Crone (wisdom) but it also honours the Horned God. These two deities are often viewed as being a sacred blend of nature (or the universe) and the Divine. The Maid-Mother-Crone symbolizes the following phases:

- **THE MAID:** Childhood and adolescence, youth and possibility, emerging sexuality;
- **THE MOTHER:** Child-bearing years, creativity, and nurturing; and
- **THE CRONE:** The menopausal years, wisdom transition, the compassion that comes from experience, and the one who guides us through the death and rebirth experience.

Each phase of the Triple-Goddess represents a different type of healing and growth in a woman's life. Her aspects are mirrored in the phases of the moon: new, waxing, full, and waning. This goddess philosophy linking spirituality and earth cycles can be found across many timeframes and cultures, including Norse, Greeks, Hindu, Celtic, and Roman belief systems.

The Mother Goddess

What specifically defines a mother goddess is the representation of her as a fertile goddess. Here are some examples of fertile goddesses from across the globe:

ALA: The Nigerian mother goddess responsible for fertility of both animals and man.

AJYST: A Siberian mother goddess whose name meant "birth giver." She visited every mother and provided a soul for the newborn.

AKA: An ancient Turkish mother goddess.

ALEMONIA: The Roman goddess responsible for the feeding of the fetus in the womb.

ARIANRHOD: A Welsh goddess associated with fertility.

AVETA: A Gallo-Roman goddess of fertility, childbirth, and midwives known mainly from clay figurines found at Toulon-sur-Allier in France.

BAST: The Egyptian cat-headed goddess associated with both fertility and childbirth.

BRIGIT: The Irish goddess of home, hearth, feminine aspects, healing, and fertility.

CORN MOTHER: The Native American goddess responsible for the fertility of the land and people.

GAIA: An ancient Greek mother goddess who gave birth to the land and the Titans.

GEFJON: One of Frigg's (Norse) handmaidens and associated with fertility of both man and the land.

HAUMEA: The Hawaiian goddess is perpetually reborn, allowing her to continually mate with her offspring.

MASTOR-AVA: A Russian earth goddess.

RAINBOW SNAKE: An Aborigine goddess representing the fertile rains and sea as she flows through her people's lives bringing children.

TLALTEUTI: The Aztec goddess of Creation. The Universe was made of her body.

VENUS: The Roman equivalent to Aphrodite and one of the main fertility goddesses.

Pregnancy And Childbirth Goddesses

ABNOBA: Gallo goddess of the Black Forest, the rivers, and childbirth.

BAST: The Egyptian cat-headed goddess associated with both childbirth and fertility.

BRIGIT: Irish deity; midwife and protector of women and children.

CANDILEFERA: The Roman goddess invoked at the beginning of childbirth. Her name means "candle bearer," and she used this light to help guide the baby into this world.

DEVERRA: The Roman goddess who protects midwives and women in birthing. Her broom was used to sweep away evil influences.

ELEITHIYA: The Greek goddess of childbirth and birthing.

FRIGG: The Nordic goddess associated with easing childbirth. A plant called Freya's grass was traditionally used as a gentle sedative during a difficult birthing.

HEKATE: The Greek midwife who carried a sacred knife to cut the cord at birth.

HEPAT: The Egyptian goddess of midwives.

ISIS: The Egyptian Goddess of many roles; protector of motherhood.

IXCHEL: The Mayan goddess of childbirth, lunar cycles, and pregnancy.

JUNO: The Roman goddess who protected pregnant woman as well as the birthing process.

MESKHENT: The Egyptian goddess who presided over the delivery of babies.

MYLITTA: The Babylonian goddess who took a special interest in the process of childbirth.

NEPHTHYS: The Egyptian goddess who stood at the head of the bed encouraging the mother whilst her sister Isis acted as midwife.

NGOLIMENTO: The Toga goddess who cared for the spirit of a child before it was born.

NINTUR: The Sumerian goddess whose name means "Lady Who Gives Form," was represented as a woman holding a midwife's pail of water.

NONA: The Roman goddess of pregnancy. Her name means "nine," relating to the ninth month of pregnancy, when the birthing woman would call upon her.

PI-HSIA-YUAN-CHUN: The Chinese goddess who protected women and children and presided over birth.

PRORSA POSTVERTA: the Roman goddess of women in birthing and associated with the position of the child in the womb.

PUKKEENEGAK: The Eskimo goddess who gives children to the Eskimo women.

SHASTI: The Indian feline goddess, depicted riding a cat. She is the goddess of childbirth and protector of children.

ST. RAYMOND NONNATUS: The Roman Catholic patron saint of midwives.

TAMAYORIHIME: The ancient Japanese sea goddess who watches over the birth waters to ensure a safe delivery.

How To Work With The Mother Goddesses

If you wish to honour the mother goddess, consider what you hope to obtain by creating a ritual. Do you want to gain something, for example, a healthy pregnancy, a natural birthing, or a profound bonding with your baby? Or do you want to show your appreciation and gratitude to the mother goddess? Learn about the different types of mother goddess, so that when you create a ritual in their name, you can do so in a way that has authentic meaning for the Divine, yourself, and your baby.

JANE'S JOURNEY

In the early days of pregnancy I struggled to actually believe that I was pregnant after such a long journey. Laurel helped me to accept through talking and exploring rituals I could do myself, that I was nurturing a new life and that my energy and self-belief was already changing. We did this through talking and creating simple rituals for me to use. Being pregnant has made me more confident in my decisions. It has also been great to increasingly think of myself as becoming part of a worldwide motherhood—a very powerful thought!

What Happens Next?

We can see that the journey through pregnancy can be full of inner symbolism. Working with this can help us to make some sense of our spiritual and psychological journey. Just as we need to learn about and nourish our inner Mother Goddess, we mustn't forget to nourish our physical body through good nutrition. The next chapter sets out recommended supplements and foods for a whole range of pregnancy symptoms.

CHAPTER 3

Good Nutrition

Good food provides not only a healthy mind and body but also supplies the raw materials your neuroendocrine (nerve-hormone) system needs to create healthy hormonal and emotional balance as you go through pregnancy.

Caution!

While there are many self-help steps you can take to improve your nutrition for the well-being of yourself and your baby, if you have any doubts or concerns about diet or supplements, consult a qualified nutritionist, your doctor or a midwife. Several US organizations provide aid to pregnant women (see Useful Resources on page 37).

Supplements

If you take vitamin supplements, make sure that they are specially formulated for pregnancy.

Folic acid

This B vitamin can reduce the risk of your baby developing spina bifida, the failure of the neural tube to close. Ideally, you should take a supplement in the first three months before conception, and then during the first three months of pregnancy, which are key times for the developing embryo.

FOR THE FOODIES: leafy green vegetables, yeast extract, fruits, and wholemeal breads and cereals.

Iron

Iron is needed to make the protein hemoglobin, which helps carry oxygen to your cells. When you are pregnant, the volume of blood in your body increases by 50 percent, requiring more hemoglobin. Later on in your pregnancy, you may need to take an iron supplement. Your iron levels will be checked during your pregnancy and, if lacking, your midwife or doctor may suggest a supplement.

FOR THE FOODIES: cocoa powder, chocolate (yippee!), tahini, broccoli, spinach, sun-dried tomatoes, chicken, parsley, turkey, roasted pumpkin and squash seeds, sunflower seeds, kale, lentils, blackstrap molasses, watercress, toasted sesame seeds, cooked egg yolks, apricots (fresh or dried), fish, red meat, haricot beans.

Calcium

Your baby needs calcium to grow bones and muscles and will take these from your body, possibly leaving you with depleted levels of calcium for yourself.

FOR THE FOODIES: yoghurt, wholewheat bread, watercress, sesame seeds, almonds, vanilla ice cream, kale, calcium-fortified milk, broccoli, rhubarb, spinach, oranges, tofu, almonds, figs, baked beans, hard cheese, fromage frais, canned sardines with bones.

What to avoid

Don't take large doses of vitamins or minerals, as this could be harmful to your baby. In particular avoid supplements that contain retinol, the animal form of vitamin A, as in large quantities, this can be toxic to unborn babies. **Tip:** The plant-based carotene type of vitamin A is safe in pregnancy.

> **WISE WOMAN WAYS**
> Talk to your doctor, midwife, or healthcare professional about special supplements you might need if you are a vegan, vegetarian, have diabetes, or have had a baby with a low birth weight before.

Gestational Diabetes

Gestational diabetes is a form of diabetes that occurs when your body can't make enough insulin to meet the extra demands of pregnancy. You're more at risk if you are:

- overweight;
- have had an unexplained miscarriage;
- are an older mum;
- have too much amniotic fluid (a colourless fluid that surrounds the baby in your uterus, protects against infection, and is involved in the development of internal organs);
- have a family history of diabetes;
- have had a previous big baby;
- or have high blood pressure.

You may have glucose in your urine, which has been detected in a routine checkup. If gestational diabetes is an issue, you'll be given information on weight control, diet, and exercise. You may be able to control your diabetes by making changes to your diet or you may need insulin injections for the remainder of your pregnancy. Any symptoms you experience will usually disappear after the birth, but you may be at higher risk of developing diabetes later in life.

For more information, contact:

Diabetes UK. *www.diabetes.org.uk*
American Diabetes Organization *www.diabetes.org/*

Foods To Avoid During Pregnancy

There are some foods that you'll need to avoid during pregnancy as they could be unsafe for your baby:

- Cheeses, such as Brie and Camembert, and blue-veined cheeses, such as Stilton. Avoid unpasteurized soft cheeses, such as those made from the milk of sheep and goats. All these cheeses could contain listeria bacteria, which can cause an infection called listeriosis that may harm your baby.
- All pâtés, meat, fish, or vegetables may contain listeria bacteria.
- Raw or undercooked meats are possible sources of bacteria that can harm your unborn baby. Make sure you cook meat thoroughly so juices run clear. Be extra careful when cooking meat on a barbecue. Make sure that meat products such as beef burgers are cooked all the way through to kill off E. coli bacteria. Chicken needs to be cooked thoroughly as it can be infected with campylobacter bacteria.
- Unpasteurized milk, and dairy products made with unpasteurized milk, aren't safe as they are likely to contain bacteria that could give you food poisoning, which you are more vulnerable to contracting during pregnancy. Pasteurized dairy products are fine.
- Peanuts and foods containing peanut products are thought to trigger a potentially serious allergy to peanuts in babies.

- Raw egg–based foods and ready-made coleslaw can contain salmonella. Throw away cracked eggs and avoid uncooked cheesecake. Cook eggs until whites and yolks are solid. Don't eat mousse, ice cream, and fresh mayonnaise when dining out as these may contain raw egg. However, salad dressings that you buy in supermarkets, such as mayonnaise, are usually made using pasteurized egg and so are safe to eat.
- Ready-made meals, including microwaveable meals, especially chicken and seafood. If you do eat them, follow cooking guidelines and serve hot to kill any harmful bacteria.
- It's best not to eat cured meats, such as Parma ham and salami, as these carry a risk of listeriosis and toxoplasmosis.
- Although oily fish is good for you and baby, it can contain environmental pollutants, so eat no more than two portions of oily fish a week. Avoid shark, swordfish, and marlin, as these contain unsafe levels of naturally occurring mercury, which can damage your baby's developing nervous system. Tuna contains some mercury, too, so it's best you don't eat more than four medium-sized cans of tuna or two fresh tuna steaks per week. Avoid raw fish, oysters, and other shellfish such as prawns—unless the prawns have been thoroughly cooked—as they may be contaminated with harmful bacteria. Safe fish includes mackerel, sardines, herrings, and pilchards.
- Avoid too much liver, liver products, and foods fortified with vitamin A, as high levels of vitamin A have been associated with birth defects.
- Stop or cut down on drinking alcohol during pregnancy.
- It's best not to have more than 200mg of caffeine a day. That's two mugs of instant coffee, four cups of black tea, or five cans of cola a day. Switch to decaffeinated hot drinks and

colas. Drinking lots of caffeine during pregnancy has been linked to low birth weight and miscarriage.

Foods To Include During Pregnancy

Your daily meals should include a variety of foods from the four main food groups:

- FRUITS AND VEGETABLES. You can buy these fresh, frozen, tinned, dried, or juiced. Aim for at least five portions (fresh or frozen) each day.
- STARCHY FOODS. These include bread, pasta, rice and potatoes. Try to choose wholegrain options for better health. Have around four servings of whole grains and carbohydrates per day, such as bread, cereals, pasta, rice, noodles, yams, and potatoes.
- PROTEIN FOODS. These include lean meat and chicken, pasteurized milk, fish, yoghurt, eggs, and pulses (such as beans and lentils). Soy products, such as tofu and miso, are a valuable source of protein. While some sources may suggest caution with soy, the National Health Service (NHS) in the United Kingdom suggests that pregnant women can eat soy products as long as they're part of a healthy, balanced diet. Try to aim for at least two portions of fish a week, including oily fish, such as sardines, herring, and wild salmon (oily fish are a good source of vitamins A and D and rich in omega-3 fatty acids) .
- DAIRY FOODS. These include milk, cheese, and yoghurt, which contain calcium. Dairy products, along with saltwater fish and unprocessed sea salt, such as Malden or Celtic sea salt, are all good sources of iodine. You need plenty of iodine in your diet to help your baby's development.

In the first few weeks of pregnancy you may not feel like eating proper meals, especially if you have nausea or sickness. However, in general you will find your body becomes more efficient when you're pregnant and makes good use of the energy you get from your food, so there is no need for extra calories during the first six months. The best rule to remember is to eat regularly. If you suffer from indigestion or heartburn, you may find that eating five or six small meals is easier on your body. Towards the end of your pregnancy, your appetite will probably increase, and for the last three months, you may find you need about an extra 200 calories per day.

> **WISE WOMAN WAYS**
>
> It's best to gain weight gradually. You'll probably gain 10kg–12.5kg (22–27.5 pounds) during your pregnancy. You may gain the least weight during the first trimester. Your weight should then steadily increase throughout the second trimester, and you may put on the most weight over the third trimester, when your baby is growing the most.

Heartburn

Heartburn can be an uncomfortable symptom during pregnancy, but it can be eased in several simple ways.

Common culprits for indigestion:
- Salt and pepper in your cooking and on your food
- White rice or flour
- Sugar in tea and coffee
- Raw salad vegetables such as onions, radishes, and cucumber
- Too much liquid, which dilutes digestive juices
- Hot, spicy food, such as curries

- Cheese just before bedtime (its high fat content slows down digestion)
- Unripe fruits (the high pectin makes them hard to digest)
- Strong tea and coffee, especially with meals
- Fatty foods or fried foods
- Pickles, sauces, and vinegar
- Bread made with wheat
- Refined foods, especially those containing sugar
- Acid-forming foods contribute to the increase of acid in our digestive system (and our body in general). These include eggs, mayonnaise, olives, fish, cranberries, bacon, beef, chicken, beans, chickpeas, lentils, pasta, lamb, prunes, Brussels sprouts, asparagus, noodles, Brazil nuts, walnuts, herrings, mackerel, rye, oats, wheat, rice, and plums.

Best foods

Ensure that 80 percent of your food consists of alkaline-forming foods, such as milk, dried fruit, almonds, coconut, beans, cabbage, celery, lettuce, avocado, mushrooms, root vegetables, bean sprouts, tomatoes, apricots, apples, banana, beetroot, raspberries, pears, peaches, melon, tangerines, oranges, lemon, grapes, grapefruit, raisins, figs, cherries, berries, rhubarb, spinach, potatoes, and carrots.

Also try the following:
- Rice cakes, oatcakes, and rye bread or spelt bread instead of wheat-based foods
- Brown rice and wholewheat bread
- Small glass of non-acidic wine as an occasional digestif
- Honey as a sweetener
- Herbal tea after meals, such as fennel, lemon verbena or mint
- Herbs in your cooking (see Chapter 4)

- Unprocessed cheese, such as mozzarella or goat's cheese, as this is a more valuable source of protein than meat as well as containing lactic acid, which aids digestion and is rich in calcium
- Stir-fried food. This is a good choice as the protein is already in smaller pieces, assisting the stomach with its function.

Have several small meals per day rather than one or two large ones and chew food thoroughly, eating slowly. This will help your body to digest your food much better.

Supplement recommendations

- DIGESTIVE ENZYMES may be helpful in supplementing your body's own digestive enzymes and assisting the breakdown of food, but they will not replace good chewing. Have a digestive enzyme (without betain hydrochloride if heartburn is present) with each main meal.
- SLIPPERY ELM herbal tea.
- GINGER has been used for colic and flatulence, as well as indigestion.
- LACTIC BACTERIA may be useful as a digestive aid by discouraging the presence of unhealthy gut bacteria.

> **WISE WOMAN WAYS**
> For an acid indigestion/heartburn remedy, dissolve one-half teaspoon of baking soda in half a glass of water and drink every two hours until the heartburn subsides.

Fatigue

Fatigue can be debilitating during pregnancy, especially in the first and third trimesters. Let's look at some ways you can help improve your energy.

Best foods

- Vitamin B sources: whole grains, organ meats e.g. heart (enjoy liver sparingly), sweet potatoes, avocados, egg yolks, fish, and whey. Both oatstraw and nettle infusions are good sources of B vitamins.
- Vitamin C sources: cantaloupe, citrus fruit and juices, kiwi, pineapple, strawberries, raspberries, broccoli, Brussels sprouts, cauliflower, green and red peppers, spinach, and tomatoes. Cooking reduces the availability of vitamin C in food, although, interestingly, cooking tomatoes increases lycopene and antioxidants, both of which can improve energy. Microwaving or steaming foods improves availability. The best food sources of vitamin C are raw fruits and vegetables.
- Tired women need more high-quality fuel, including good fats, in their diet, especially natural sources of vitamin E, such as avocados, peanut butter, sunflower seeds, tahini, and olive oil. Herbs rich in vitamin E include nettle, seaweeds, dandelion, and watercress.
- Celery, cabbage, seaweeds, nettle infusion, and red clover infusion are excellent sources of potassium.
- For iodine, consume seaweeds, unprocessed sea salt, mushrooms, and leafy greens grown in gardens fertilized with seaweed.
- You may need to increase your intake of iron. Consume a spoonful of blackstrap molasses or take a dropper of yellow

dock tincture several times a day. Chocolate, seaweeds, nettle infusion, and dandelion leaves are also superb sources of iron.

The following foods are naturally high in vitamins and minerals and will help you sustain energy throughout the day:

- Peanut butter and almond butter
- Live-culture yoghurt
- Slightly underripe banana
- Cheese and oatcakes
- Turkey breast sandwich
- Hard-boiled egg
- Chicken salad on wholewheat pita bread
- Pasta salad
- Baked potato with low-fat cheese topping

Water Retention

Water retention, or edema, can make a pregnant woman look and feel like a balloon. Here are a few tips on lessening the water in your body.

Best foods

- Foods that relieve water retention include asparagus, nettles, corn (and corn silk tea), grapes, cucumbers, watermelon (and watermelon seed tea), parsley, celery, black tea and green tea (no more than four cups a day).
- Avoid eating too much regular salt.

Constipation

Constipation can be uncomfortable while in our body—and also when coming out! Let's look at how we might keep things moving along in the body.

Best foods

- If you need an iron supplement because you are prone to anemia, try Floradix or a liquid iron supplement (check with your midwife first).
- Eat extra red meat and dark green vegetables.
- Start your day with a cup of warm water with a slice of lemon in it.
- Start each meal with salad or fruit, and eat lots of foods that are high in fibre (roughage) and vitamin C.
- Fresh fruits, such as oranges, grapefruits, tangerines, black-currants, dried prunes, and apricots, and vegetables, including celery, watercress, cabbage, spinach, and artichokes, are all good, as are wholegrain cereals and bread.
- Beans, lentils, and pulses are other useful high-fibre foods.
- Psyllium or ispagula husks, the seeds from plantain, have been shown in some research to be effective for constipation, particularly in those with irritable bowel syndrome.
- I always recommend linseed (flax seed), which are rich in fibre and essential fatty acids, to pregnant women suffering from constipation.
- A high-fibre diet provides more roughage, which helps with digestion, but remember to increase your fluid intake to at least 1.5 litres (2.6 pints) of water daily.
- Avoid drinks that function as a diuretic (make you pass more urine), such as black tea, coffee, cola, and alcohol, as these can dehydrate you, making constipation worse.

If you use bran to manage constipation increase your fluid intake, as without extra water, bran will make your stool hard and difficult to pass through the intestines.

WISE WOMAN WAYS

This might not be dinner party reading, but the information may help you manage your bowel movements better. When you are sitting, your puborectalis muscle restricts your rectum in order to maintain "continence." This leads to the anal canal not being straight, which can result in unfinished or constrictive bowel movements when on the loo. However, a relaxed, full-squat posture (useful practice for birthing!) relaxes the puborectalis muscle and straightens the rectum, leading to a better bowel movement. Some useful sites for toilet-squatting products: *www.naturesplatform.com* or *www.toilet-related-ailments.com/index.html.*

Pregnancy Sickness

Pregnancy sickness can make life pretty miserable. It's often a case of just getting through it. Here are some tips that might help.

Best foods

- Eat a small slice of orange or grapefruit.
- Adding a little lemon to your drinking water may also help relieve your symptoms of pregnancy sickness.
- If you can't stand the smell of cooked food, make yourself a nutritious smoothie or try juicing using only fresh fruits and vegetables. This way you will keep yourself hydrated and well nourished. If you have a juicer, you can try a combination of pineapple, apple, carrot, and ginger.
- Sucking on crushed ice could help keep the nausea at bay.
- I've had women tell me raspberries are helpful.
- Make an infusion tea from freshly crushed or grated ginger root and drink it ever so often. Or try peppermint tea.

JANE'S JOURNEY

Constipation is one of the symptoms of pregnancy that I wasn't aware of until it happened! Laurel has helped me with this by recommending I eat dates and use cracked golden linseed on cereal in salads and stir-frys. It worked wonders! Another bit of advice, which worked for nausea, was to eat little and often. I remember we talked about the importance of complex carbs and protein snacking to improve energy. The second trimester brought even more fatigue, so I increased iron-based foods. (I went on to take liquid iron as well.)

What Happens Next?

A nourishing diet during pregnancy will help our bodies deal with the changing hormones. As Wise Women, we also know the value of using herbs as part of our daily nutrition. I cover this in the next chapter.

Useful Resources

Organizations

- British Association for Applied Nutrition and Nutritional Therapy, *www.bant.org.uk* (for listings of qualified nutritional therapists)
- American Dietetic Association, *www.eatright.org* (for registered dieticians)
- Department of Health (US): The Special Supplemental Nutrition Program (SNAP) for Women, Infants and Children (WIC) offers nutrition education, breastfeeding support, referrals, and a variety of nutritious foods to low-income pregnant, breastfeeding or postpartum women, infants, and children up to age five to promote and support good health. *www.health.ny.gov/prevention/nutrition/wic*

- Commodity Supplemental Food Program (US): CSFP works to improve the health of low-income pregnant and breastfeeding women, other new mothers up to one year postpartum, infants and children up to age six by supplementing their diets with nutritious USDA commodity foods. *www.fns.usda.gov/fdd/programs/csfp*
- NHS (UK). Pregnancy care. *www.nhs.uk/Planners/pregnancycareplanner/Pages/Eating.aspx*

Supplements

- The Nutri Centre, *www.nutricentre.com*

CHAPTER 4

Wort Cunning

The Wise Woman going through pregnancy will embrace the use of herbs (ideally organic) into her healing regime. It is important to note that not all herbs are beneficial for pregnant women. Please consult a qualified herbalist before taking herbs.

Caution!

While there are many safe herbs you can take to improve the well-being of yourself and your baby, if you have any doubts or concerns about which herbs are safe, consult a qualified herbalist.

Useful Herbs During Pregnancy

Several herbs safely used by pregnant women for generations can easily be made into teas and incorporated into meals on a regular basis:

NETTLE LEAVES have a high iron and calcium content and are a good source of folic acid. They strengthen the kidneys and adrenals and relieve fluid retention. Because nettle also supports the vascular system, it can prevent varicose veins and piles. Postpartum, it increases breast milk.

> **WISE WOMAN WAYS**
> Cooked nettle is a mineral-rich substitute for spinach. Pick it fresh (from places which are not affected from pesticides such as roadsides) from spring until mid-summer, wearing gloves to protect your skin. Ensure you pick the herbs in places where they are not sprayed with pesticides.

Boil young nettle leaves in a closed saucepan with a small amount of water or stock for about 4 minutes. Strain off the water (you can use this as a hair rinse at a later stage) and press the nettles slightly through a sieve to remove excess water. Serve the boiled nettle leaves with a knob of butter and a generous twist of black pepper or lemon juice and sesame seeds.

OATS are high in calcium and magnesium, build healthy bones, nourish the nervous system, and allow good sleep. An easy way to incorporate oats into your diet is to eat hot porridge (whole steelcut oats or pinhead oats are best) for breakfast in the morning, along with oatmeal bread or oatcakes. **Tip:** A warm oatmeal bath softens skin and relieves the itch of a growing belly.

DANDELION ROOT TEA increases digestion and promotes bile to relieve constipation. It is one of the best herbs for cleansing and strengthening the body's main detoxifying organ: the liver. (In addition, the liver breaks down hormones no longer needed by the body after birth, as well as any drugs that may have been given prior to delivery). Add a handful of fresh dandelion leaves to salads. Drink dandelion leaf tea for a natural diuretic, or try roasted dandelion root (with iron and calcium) as a coffee substitute.

ALFALFA, with its deep root system, contains many essential nutrients, including trace minerals, chlorophyll, and vitamin K, a nutrient necessary for blood clotting. Many midwives advise drinking mild-tasting alfalfa tea or taking alfalfa tablets during the last trimester of pregnancy to decrease postpartum bleeding or the chance of hemorrhaging. Alfalfa also increases breast milk.

Herbs To Avoid During Pregnancy

To ensure you take only safe herbs for you and your baby, consult a qualified herbalist. The following herbs and substances should be avoided:

- ALOE VERA stimulates uterine contractions. Avoid when breastfeeding.
- ARBOR VITAE causes uterine surges.
- AUTUMN CROCUS can affect cell division and lead to birth defects.
- BARBERRY is known to stimulate uterine surges.
- BASIL OIL is a uterine stimulant. Use only during birthing.
- BLACK COHOSH can cause premature surges but is safe during birthing.
- BLUE COHOSH is a uterine stimulant but is safe during birthing.
- CAFFEINE can cause high blood pressure.
- COMFREY contains toxic chemicals that could cross the placenta.
- COTTON ROOT is a uterine stimulant.
- CUMIN SEED/POWDER can cause premature birthing, miscarriage, or cramping.
- DONG QUAI is a menstrual stimulant and can bring on strong surges.
- FALSE UNICORN ROOT may cause nausea and vomiting.
- FEVERFEW is a uterine stimulant.
- GOLDENSEAL may lead to premature birthing or miscarriage but is safe during birthing.
- JUNIPER/JUNIPER OIL are uterine stimulants but can be used during birthing.

- LICORICE can cause high blood pressure.
- MUGWORT may lead to birth defects. Avoid when breast-feeding.
- PENNYROYAL can cause birth defects. Avoid when breast-feeding.
- PERUVIAN BARK is highly toxic and can cause coma, blindness, or even death.
- POKE ROOT may cause birth defects.
- RUE is a menstrual stimulant that may cause premature surges.
- SASSAFRAS is a uterine stimulant and may also cause birth defects.
- SHEPHERD'S PURSE is a uterine stimulant. Use only during birthing.
- TANSY is a uterine stimulant and may cause birth defects.
- WILD YAM is a uterine stimulant but is safe during birthing.
- WORMWOOD may cause birth defects. Avoid when breast-feeding.

Constipation

Constipation is common in pregnancy because the hormone progesterone relaxes and slows down the movement of your intestines. Additionally, as pregnancy progresses and your baby gets bigger, increased downward pressure increases pelvic congestion, making constipation more likely. It is important to prevent constipation as it can make hemorrhoids (piles) worse. **Tip:** Liquid Floridix is fabulous and doesn't bung you up.

Here are some things to try:

Herbal Remedies

DANDELION or MALLOW TEA, made from the leaves of the plants, steeped in boiling water and drunk daily can help treat constipation.

Aromatherapy

Add three to four drops of essential oils such as SWEET ORANGE, LEMON, LIME, GRAPEFRUIT, OR BERGAMOT to your bath and relax in the warm water for a while; you could also use plenty of soap lather to massage your tummy gently in a clockwise direction. Avoid very firm massage, especially if you have had any threat of premature birth or if your placenta is lying low in your uterus.

> **WISE WOMAN WAYS**
> Staying active can help prevent constipation. Swimming (have a go at aquanatal classes!), tai chi, walking, qi gong, cycling, pregnancy yoga, or other more formal pregnancy exercise classes can all help to keep the bowels moving.

Pregnancy Sickness

GINGER ROOT TEA can help if the nausea is constant. Prepare a tea with fresh-grated ginger root and sip throughout the day to alleviate persistent nausea. **Note:** do not take excessive amounts of ginger during pregnancy as eating more than 1g a day may cause birth defects and other problems (according to *www.MayoClinic.com*).

PEPPERMINT TEA can be taken any time, but it is very useful if taken upon waking.

Water Retention

- CLEAVERS is especially helpful for swollen, sore breasts.
- EVENING PRIMROSE OIL is an adaptogen (a substance that is safe, increases resistance to stress, and has a balancing effect on body functions) and is useful for fluid retention.

Headaches

- Chinese herbalists say headaches are caused by liver stress. Liver-strengthening herbs are DANDELION, YELLOW DOCK, MILKTHISTLE SEED, and BURDOCK.
- SAGE offers relief from headaches.
- SKULLCAP can ease pain and relieve muscle spasms.
- EVENING PRIMROSE OIL is useful for headaches.

Insomnia

- OATSTRAW promotes sound sleep.

Fatigue

- OATSTRAW builds energy and eases anxiety.
- NETTLE increases energy without wiring your nerves and strengthens the adrenals, allowing you to tolerate more stress with less harm. The plants that are deepest green in colour give you the most energy. Drink a daily cup of nettle infusion for fatigue.
- SARSAPARILLA can increase energy and overall feelings of vitality.

Herbal Sources Of Vitamins

- VITAMIN B COMPLEX: For healthy digestion, emotional flexibility, less anxiety, and sound sleep. Depleted by hormone replacement treatment (HRT). *Herbal sources:* Oatstraw.

- VITAMIN B1 (THIAMINE): For emotional ease, strong nerves. *Herbal sources:* Peppermint, burdock, sage, yellow dock, alfalfa, raspberry leaves, nettle, watercress, and rose buds and hips.
- VITAMIN B2 (RIBOFLAVIN): For more energy and healthy skin. Depleted by hot flushes. *Herbal sources:* Peppermint, alfalfa greens, echinacea, yellow dock, hops, dandelion root, dulse, kelp, rose hips, and nettles.
- VITAMIN B9 (FOLIC ACID): For calm nerves. *Herbal sources:* Leafy greens of nettles, alfalfa, sage, peppermint, plantain, comfrey, and chickweed.
- VITAMIN B3 (NIACIN): For relief of anxiety and depression and a decrease in headaches. *Herbal sources:* Hops, raspberry leaf, red clover; slippery elm, echinacea, rose hips, nettle, and alfalfa.
- BIOFLAVONOIDS: For a healthy heart and to reduce water retention, and anxiety. *Herbal sources:* Buckwheat greens, elderberries, hawthorn fruits, rose hips, horsetail, shepherd's purse, and chervil.
- CAROTENES: For a well-lubricated vagina, strong bones, and healthy lungs and skin. *Herbal sources:* Peppermint, yellow dock, uva ursi, alfalfa, raspberry, nettles, dandelion greens, kelp, green onions, violet leaves, cayenne, paprika, lamb's quarters leaves, sage, chickweed, horsetail, and rose hips.
- VITAMIN C COMPLEX: For relief from insomnia, reduces headaches and promotes easier emotions. Also useful when you are depleted from too much stress. *Herbal sources:* Rose hips, yellow dock root, raspberry leaf, hops, pine needles, dandelion greens, alfalfa greens, echinacea, skullcap, plantain, cayenne, and paprika.

- VITAMIN E: For fewer signs of aging and a moist vagina. *Herbal sources:* Alfalfa, rosehips, nettles, watercress, dandelion, seaweeds, wild seeds of lamb's quarters, and plantain.
- ESSENTIAL FATTY ACIDS (EFAS), INCLUDING GLA, OMEGA-6, and OMEGA-3: For a healthy heart, strong nerves, well-functioning endocrine glands, and fewer wrinkles. All wild plants, but very few cultivated plants, contain EFAs; fresh purslane is notably high.
- VITAMIN K: For stronger bones. *Herbal sources:* Nettle, alfalfa, kelp, green tea.

WISE WOMAN WAYS

Herbal honeys are made by pouring honey over fresh herbs and allowing them to merge over a period of several days to several months. As the herbs are infused with honey, the water-loving honey absorbs all the water-soluble and anti-infective volatile oils of the herb. Here's how to create your herbal honey:

- Coarsely chop the dried herb of your choice (ginger and garlic should be used fresh). You could use sage, rose, mint, oregano, lemon verbena, lavender, thyme, rosemary, marjoram, or lemon balm.
- Put chopped herb into a wide-mouthed jar, filling almost to the top.
- Pour pasteurized honey into the jar, working it into the herb with a wooden spoon.
- Fill the jar to the very top and cover tightly and label.

Your herbal honey is ready to use in as little as a day or two, but will be more medicinal if allowed to sit for six weeks. Use your herbal honey by spreading it on homemade bread or placing a tablespoonful (include herb as well as honey) into a mug of boiling water.

Herbal Sources Of Minerals

- BORON: For strong, flexible bones. *Herbal sources:* All organic garden weeds, including all edible parts of chickweed, purslane, nettles, dandelion, and yellow dock.
- CALCIUM: For sound sleep, freedom from depression and headaches, less bloating, and fewer mood fluctuations. *Herbal sources:* Valerian, kelp, nettle, horsetail, peppermint; sage, uva ursi, yellow dock, chickweed, oatstraw, black currant leaf, raspberry leaf, plantain leaf/seed, dandelion leaf, amaranth leaf/seed, and lamb's quarter leaf/seed.
- CHROMIUM: For less fatigue, fewer mood swings, and stable blood sugar levels. *Herbal sources:* Oatstraw, nettle, dulse, wild yam, horsetail, echinacea, valerian, as well as sarsaparilla.
- COPPER: For supple skin, healthy hair, calm nerves, and less water retention. *Herbal sources:* Skullcap, sage, horsetail, and chickweed.
- IODINE: For less fatigue. *Herbal sources:* Kelp and sarsaparilla root.
- IRON: For fewer headaches, better sleep, calmer nerves, and more energy. *Herbal sources:* Chickweed, kelp, burdock root, horsetail, Althea root, milk thistle seed, uva ursi, dandelion leaf/root; yellow dock, echinacea, valerian, and sarsaparilla roots; and nettles, plantain leaf, and peppermint.
- MAGNESIUM: For deeper sleep, less anxiety, easier nerves, and fewer headaches/migraines. *Herbal sources:* Oatstraw, kelp, nettle, dulse, burdock root, chickweed, Althea root, horsetail, sage, raspberry leaf, valerian, yellow dock, dandelion greens, carrot tops, and evening primrose.
- MANGANESE: For flexible bones. *Herbal sources:* Raspberry, uva ursi leaf, chickweed, milk thistle seed, yellow dock;

ginseng, wild yam, echinacea, and dandelion roots; and
nettle, kelp, horsetail, and hops flowers.

- MOLYBDENUM: For prevention of anemia. *Herbal sources:* Nettles, dandelion greens, sage, oatstraw, raspberry leaves, horsetail, chickweed, and kelp.
- NICKEL: For calmer nerves. *Herbal sources:* Alfalfa and oatstraw.
- PHOSPHORUS: For strong, flexible bones and more energy. *Herbal sources:* Peppermint, yellow dock, milk thistle, fennel, hops, chickweed, nettle, dandelion, and dulse.
- POTASSIUM: For more energy, less fatigue, less water retention, and better digestion. *Herbal sources:* Sage, peppermint, skullcap, hops, dulse, kelp, horsetail, nettles, and plantain leaf.
- SELENIUM: For slower aging, strong immunity, less irritability, more energy, healthy hair/nails/teeth, and less cardiovascular disease. *Herbal sources:* Milk thistle seed, valerian root, dulse, uva ursi leaf, hops flowers, kelp, raspberry leaf, rose buds and hips, hawthorn berries, roots of echinacea, sarsaparilla, and yellow dock.
- SILICON: For strong, flexible bones, less irritable nerves. *Herbal sources:* Horsetail, dulse, echinacea, cornsilk, burdock, oatstraw, chickweed, uva ursi, and sarsaparilla.
- SULPHUR: For soft skin, glossy hair, and healthy nerves. *Herbal sources:* Sage, nettles, plantain, and horsetail.
- ZINC: For better digestion, healthy skin, and increased sex drive. *Herbal sources:* Skullcap, sage, wild yam, chickweed, echinacea, nettles, dulse, milk thistle, and sarsaparilla.

WISE WOMAN WAYS

Consult a qualified herbalist before taking any herbs while pregnant or if you are on ANY medication.

What Happens Next?

The use of herbs in Wise Woman healing, both internally and externally, is part of our sacred heritage. While flower essences aren't to be confused with herbs or essential oils, they too have their precious place in our life during pregnancy. Read on to discover how you might use these gifts from nature.

Useful Resources

Organizations

National Institute for Medical Herbalists, *www.nimh.org.uk*
American Herbalists Guild, *www.americanherbalistsguild.com*

CHAPTER 5

Using Flower Essences
for Pregnancy

From the beginning of time, nature has provided the means to heal on all levels. Flower essences have been used for centuries in Australia, South America, Asia, Egypt, South America, and India. They were also very popular in Europe in the Middle Ages. Hildegard von Bingen, a 12th-century visionary who wrote medicinal texts, and Paracelsus, a 15th-century physician and astrologer, both wrote how they used dew collected from flowering plants to treat health imbalances.

How Flower Essences Work

Flower essences are a form of vibrational medicine and act in a similar way to homeopathic remedies by working with subtle energy in the body. All living things, including our body and mind, are matter that is permeated by, and surrounded by subtle energy. We could define subtle energy as the underpinning source feeding the well-being of our mind and body.

According to the concept of energy medicine, disease manifests in the physical body only after energy flow in the subtle body has been disturbed. Energy medicine has long been practised by civilizations such as India and China, and is gradually being integrated into Western healthcare. The energy field model used by these civilizations as part of their eclectic healthcare system, which includes acupuncture, moves away from the main idea that life evolves from a scientific blueprint towards the concept that life circulates via electrical charges of energy known as *prana* or *chi*.

In addition to this circulation of energy, there is a force field of energy permeating the human body called the aura, which can influence our well-being. In order to rebalance the subtle body, we must administer energy that vibrates at frequencies beyond the physical plane. Just as we might heal the physical body through medical interventions, we need to heal the subtle body through vibrational interventions such as homeopathy, crystals, or flower essences.

Flower essences work by utilizing the essence's positive energy to transmute a negative state in living things, whether they are human, animal, or plant. Each flower used in a flower essence conveys a subtle energy pattern that is transferred to water during essence preparation. This preparation is then either used internally or externally for healing purposes.

From a spiritual perspective, flower essences address mental and emotional imbalances that, if left unresolved, could influence the wellness of the physical body. In effect, we "co-create" with the flower essences to alter our subtle energies when we use them for healing purposes. This change permeates our emotional and mental states and can also influence our physical well-being. The belief that we can heal ourselves is the basis of flower essence philosophy.

Essences do not affect us biochemically, as does traditional allopathic medicine. They are water-based products that have no chemical or biological materials present other than the water and alcohol preservatives they are prepared in.

Bach Flower Remedies

Dr. Edward Bach studied medicine at University College Hospital, London, qualified in 1912, and became casualty medical officer at the hospital in 1913. He worked in general practice in London's famed medical sector Harley Street and as a bacteriologist and pathologist working on vaccines. In the course of his work, he came to question some of the tenets of early

20th-century medical practice. Bach believed that the illness-personality link was a product of unbalanced energetic patterns within the subtle body, and that illness was a reflection of disharmony between the physical personality and the Higher Self.

Bach took a post at the Royal London Homeopathic Hospital (1919), where he noticed the parallels between his work on vaccines and the principles of homeopathy. Although his work up to this point had been with bacteria, he wanted to find healing modalities that would be less toxic and more in tune with the mind-body link. To this end, he began collecting plants in the hope of replacing the nosodes (homeopathic remedies prepared from infected tissues) with a series of gentler remedies.

In 1928, Bach acquired two wildflowers, impatiens and mimulus, which he homeopathically prepared and clinically used with excellent results. He soon understood that there was great healing power in flowers, and he gradually developed his own methods of preparing flower essences. In the early 1930s, Bach left his successful practice and began gathering more wildflowers, which he developed into 38 flower remedies.

Instead of scientific methodology, he chose to rely on his intuitive gifts as a healer. He found that he could place the flowers of a particular species on the surface of a bowl of spring water for several hours in sunlight and obtain powerful vibrational tinctures. The subtle effects of sunlight charged the water with an energetic imprint of the flower's unique signature. In 1934, Dr. Bach moved to Mount Vernon in Oxfordshire, England, and it was here, in the surrounding countryside, that he found the remaining flower remedies he sought, each aimed at a particular mental state or emotion. Bach's work was in tune with nature's own annual cycle. In spring and summer, he found the flowers he needed in the countryside and prepared individual flower remedies, then in winter, he helped and advised patients. He found that when he treated the feelings of his patients, their distress and physical discomfort would be alleviated to allow their natural healing to come through.

The 38 Bach Flower Remedies include:

agrimony	aspen
beech	centaury
cerato	cherry plum
chestnut bud	chicory
clematis	crab apple
elm	gentian
gorse	heather
holly	honeysuckle
hornbeam	impatiens
larch	mimulus
mustard	oak
olive	pine
red chestnut	rock rose
rock water	schleranthus
star of Bethlehem	sweet chestnut
vervain	vine
walnut	water violet
white chestnut	wild oat
wild rose	willow

Pregnancy State	Recommended Bach Flower Remedy
Pregnancy sickness	crab apple, scleranthus
Difficulty in accepting pregnancy	willow, walnut
Fear; of birthing, pain, becoming a parent	mimulus, rock rose
Mood changes	scleranthus

Impatience	impatiens
Feeling overwhelmed	elm
Worry, apprehension	white chestnut, red chestnut, aspen, and larch
Feeling like an elephant!	crab apple
Depression	cherry plum, gentian, gorse, mustard, white chestnut, and wild rose
Fretful	agrimony
Fuzzy thinking, lack of concentration	crab apple, clematis
Indecisive, self-doubting	cerato, scleranthus, wild oat
Insomnia	holly, hornbeam, mustard, olive, white chestnut
Intolerant, critical, irritable	beech, holly, impatiens, rock water, vervain, vine, crab apple
Irrational without knowing why	cherry plum
Lack of confidence	centaury, larch, and mimulus
Lack of sexual interest	clematis
Overburdened	hornbeam, olive
Panic	cherry plum, rock rose
Procrastination	hornbeam
Resentful	willow
Uncomfortable/ ashamed of body	crab apple
Tired, drained	olive
Headache	aspen, vervain, white chestnut
Dizziness	aspen, clematis
Leg cramps	impatiens

I came to the Bach Flower Remedies about 25 years ago. A friend had a computer and photocopy shop, and I would sometimes help out. One day a nutritionist came in with a mound of copying to do, much of it related to flower essences. Being full of curiosity, I was reading as I was copying. It was like coming home. I learnt the remedies by using them on myself, and since those days all the remedies have been in my home ready to use with family, friends, animals, plants, clients, students, and myself.

Animals and young children respond particularly well to Bach Flower Remedies. I remember going to an animal sanctuary on the request of a student of mine who worked there. In a glass terrarium was a mother snake and several babies. Mum snake, bless her, had a cold and was coiled in a corner. I made up a remedy for the student to give to the mother snake, and within minutes she picked up and got right into a bit of family entwining! I've given remedies to cats following operations and dogs in crisis over fireworks on Guy Fawkes Night in November.

I've also had lots of success giving remedies to babies and young children with sleep and behavioural issues, at the parent's request. I've found that it's important to use the remedy or remedies that resonate as the right ones at the gut level—however off the wall they might seem at the time. It's a good idea to carry Bach Flower Rescue Remedy as an emergency stress-buster. It's a mixture of rock rose, impatiens, clematis, star of Bethlehem, and cherry plum and works rapidly to calm the body.

Australian Bush Flower Essences

Since Dr. Bach created his flower essences in the 1930s, the issues we face in our lives have changed. As we came to the end of the 20th century and slipped into the 21st century, there was a growing need for flower essences that help people deal with the issues of today.

While many new flower essences have found their way to the commercial market, some of the most effective new flower essences come from Australian plants as a result of the work of Ian White, a naturopath and fifth-generation Australian herbalist. Ian grew up in the Australian bush. As a young boy his grandmother, like her mother before her, specialized in using Australian plants and would often take him bush walking to learn the healing qualities of plants and flowers. He learned a profound respect for nature through her and went on to become a practitioner and a pioneer working with and researching the rare remedial qualities of Australian native plants. Australia is relatively unpolluted, has some of the world's oldest plants, and metaphysically has a wise, old energy.

The 65 Australian Bush Essences include:

alpine mint bush	angelsword
banksia robur	bauhinia
billy goat plum	black-eyed Susan
bluebell	boab
boronia	bottlebrush
bush fuchsia	bush gardenia
bush iris	crowea
dagger hakea	dog rose
dog rose of wild forces	five corners
flannel flower	fresh water mangrove
fringed violet	green spider orchid
grey spider flower	gymea lily
hibbertia	illawarra flame tree
isopogon	jacaranda
kangaroo paw	kapok bush
little flannel flower	macrocarpa
mint bush	mountain devil
mulla mulla	old man banksia
paw paw	peach-flowered tea tree

philotheca
red grevillea
red lily
rough bluebell
silver princess
Southern Crosss
sturt desert pea
sundew
tall mulla mulla
turkey bush
wedding bush
wisteria

pink mulla mulla
red helmet orchid
red suva frangipani
she oak
slender rice flower
pinifex
sturt desert rose
sunshine wattle
tall yellow top
waratah
wild potato bush
yellow cowslip orchid

Pregnancy State	Recommended Australian Bush Essence
Apprehensive, anxious	tall mulla mulla, dog rose, illawarra flame tree
Shock of unplanned pregnancy	fringed violet
Constipation	bauhinia, bottlebrush, flannel flower, bluebell
Depression	waratah, tall yellow top
Self-doubting	five corners, kapok bush, red grevillea, bush fuchsia
Insomnia	boronia, grey spider flower, black-eyed susan, and crowea
Intolerant, critical, irritable	yellow cowslip orchid, mountain devil, and black-eyed Susan
Lack of confidence	five corners, kapok bush
Lack of sexual interest	billy goat plum
Managing change	bauhinia, bottlebrush, mint bush, pink mulla mulla, and silver princess

Mental and emotional exhaustion	alpine mint bush, banksia robur, macrocarpa
Panic	grey spider flower, dog rose of the wild forces
Resentful	dagger hakea
Uncomfortable, ashamed of body	billy goat plum, wild potato bush, wisteria, spinifex
Tired, drained	old man banksia
Worry	crowea
Bonding with baby	bottlebrush
Post-partum overwhelm	bottlebrush, she oak, tallyellow top, dog rose of the wild forces, waratah, illawarra flame tree
Acidity	crowea
Anemia	bluebell, five corners, kapokbush, red grevillea, waratah
High blood pressure	bluebell, crowea, five corners, hibbertia, little flannel flower, mountain devil, mulla mulla
Premature childbirth	fringed violet, sturt desert rose, sunshine wattle, waratah
Leg cramps	black-eyed susan, bottlebrush, crowea, and grey spider
Dizziness	bush fuscia, crowea
Sinusitis	bush iris, dagger hakea, fringed violet
Physical exhaustion	marcrocarpa
Headache	black-eyed susan
Pregnancy memory (or lack of it!)	isopogon

The Australian Bush Flower Essences found me through a book—or rather that's how I remembered them again. While I have never been to Australia, there is some link to this wild country in my soul. I've used them increasingly over the years. I have the full range of bush essences, which I often blend with the Bach Flower Remedies. I find the Australian Bush Flower Essences very profound in their action.

> **WISE WOMAN WAYS**
>
> When using flower essences, it's important to use them in an integrated way. Don't just take them mindlessly. When I take a remedy, I consider why I'm taking it and what I can do to support myself in other ways. For example, if I'm taking a mixture for anger, I ask myself what or who my anger is directed at. What can I do to help externalize this feeling? What is it about? I might choose to journal my thoughts and feelings or talk them through with someone, taking the remedies as I consciously work through my issue.

How To Mix And Use Remedies

Here are a variety of ways you can use the remedies:

Combination mixtures

Using a blend of Bach Flower Essences and Australia Bush Essences, you can make up these remedies. Take them either directly from the bottle or moisten your lips. **Note:** BF = Bach Flowers and ABFE = Australian Bush Flower Essences

Pregnancy State	Recommended Remedy
Pregnancy sickness	Take these four ABFE together: dog rose, paw paw, dagger hakea, crowea

Fear of birthing pain	mimulus (BF), rock rose (BF)
Impatience	impatiens (BF)
Feeling overwhelmed	elm (BF)
Worry	white chestnut (BF), red chestnut (BF), aspen (BF), larch (BF), tall mulla mulla (ABFE), dog rose (ABFE), illawarra flame tree (ABFE), crowea (ABFE), agrimony (BF)
Lack of confidence	centaury (BF), larch (BF), mimulus (BF), five corners (ABFE), kapok bush (ABFE)
Panic	cherry plum (BF), rock rose (BF), grey spider flower (ABFE), dog rose of the wild forces (ABFE)
Tired, drained	olive (BF), old man banksia (ABFE), marcrocarpa (ABFE)
Self-doubting	five corners (ABFE), kapok bush (ABFE), red grevillea (ABFE), cerato (BF), wild oat (BF)
Mental and emotional exhaustion	alpine mint bush (ABFE), banksia robur (ABFE), macrocarpa (ABFE)
Post-partum overwhelm	bottlebrush (ABFE), she oak (ABFE), tall yellow top (ABFE), dog rose of thewild forces (ABFE), waratah (ABFE) Anxietyaspen (BF), mimulus (BF), larch (BF), rock rose (BF), crowea (ABFE), illawarra flame tree (ABFE)
Irritability	beech (BF), vervain (BF),black-eyed susan (ABFE), yellow cowslip orchid (ABFE)

Internal

Bach Flower and Australian Bush Flower Essences can be taken orally for acute cases by putting two or three drops of the stock bottle essence under the tongue. They can be taken longer-term by taking six drops from a dropper bottle that contains stock essence plus water. To make up a remedy:

1. Fill a 20ml glass dropper bottle with tap or filtered water to a finger width beneath the neck of the bottle.
2. Choose your remedy (you can use a mixture of Australian Bush Flower Essences and Bach Flower Remedies for up to six remedies). Drop two drops from the stock bottle into the dropper bottle.
3. If you are a Reiki practitioner, you might like to perform Reiki on the bottle.
4. Take four drops under the tongue, four times daily. Alternatively you can put the remedies in tea, coffee, fizzy drinks, and so on. If you are taking a made-up remedy, you might have four drops, four times daily for a period of one month or lunar cycle.
   Note: Putting the drops into a hot drink has the advantage of evaporating the alcohol. This is sometimes recommended to people who dislike the alcohol content or who are too sensitive to alcohol to take remedies containing it, such as those with adrenal issues.

Because of the dynamic nature of awakening and going to sleep at night, the most important times to take the remedy is immediately upon waking and before going to sleep. The other two times may be before lunch and around 6pm.

- INHALING: Put two drops of your chosen essence in the palm of your hands, rub them together and inhale from them.
- MEDITATION: One of the most powerful ways to use the essences is to take a few drops just before meditating.
- IN FOOD: When you make nourishing food for yourself and your baby, add your remedy to the food, either straight from the stock bottle or from your dropper bottle mixture.

WISE WOMAN WAYS

I find that taking the remedies is a multilayered opportunity for personal growth. When I feel distressed, I want the feelings to go away. I don't like feeling uncomfortable. I want to feel good. However, it isn't helpful to use the remedies as a "Band-Aid." Yes, the feelings may ease, but they may return again. Let's use anxiety as an example. Very often anxiety is the "acceptable face" we show the world. Anxiety, however, often covers up a range of other emotions that maybe aren't quite as "acceptable." Only the other day, I experienced feelings of being overwhelmed and anxious due to external pressures. I took myself off, did some relaxation exercises, a few stretches, and screamed into a cushion for good measure. There was the anger my anxiety had been holding down. So I took a remedy for the anger and helped myself through the blip.

External

- COMPRESS: This can be useful, especially where there is a sore place, such as breasts or lower back, and during birthing. To prepare a flower essence compress, fill a bowl with warm or cold water. Add four drops of each chosen flower essence (and one or two drops of appropriate essential oil if you like) to the water. Soak the washcloth in the water, wring out and lay it on the affected area and repeat until relief is felt.

WISE WOMAN WAYS

If your boobs feel tender, sprinkle several drops of she oak on a damp, cool washcloth and place on the sensitive area to bring relief.

- BATHING: Run a bath. The water needs to be at body temperature or a little warmer. Add one or two drops of your chosen flower essence. Essential oils can also be added after the water is run. Get into the bath and relax for 20 minutes (remember this one during your birthing). Rest well afterwards. If you don't want to have a full bath, bathing the feet and/or hands is also an effective way to take essences in through the skin.
- BODY SPRAY: Adding essential oils to a body spray not only brings healing benefits but also a wonderful, uplifting smell. Lighter oils such as lavender or lemongrass work best for this purpose.

  To prepare a flower essence spray, fill a 50-125ml glass spray bottle with springwater. Add three or four drops of essential oil. Add three drops of each chosen flower essence. Shake the bottle to activate the essences and spray twice daily, or as required. This would be a good idea for your birthing kit.
- CHAKRA POINTS: With just a little knowledge of the chakra system, the seven wheel-shaped energy centers in the body, you can apply flower essences to a chakra area either directly from the stock bottle or take internally:

Chakra	Recommended Australian and Bach Flower Remedies
FIRST: Root (base)	Waratah, red lily (disconnection), sundew (indecisive), grey spider (panic), macrocarpa (exhaustion), rock rose (panic), clematis (ungrounded), hornbeam (mental exhaustion)
SECOND: Sacral (spleen)	Turkey bush (creativity), billy goat plum (releases shame), spinifex (cleansing), she oak (hormonal imbalance)
THIRD: Solar plexus	Old man banksia (counteracts weariness), macrocarpa (energy), crowea (releases worry), wild potato bush (releases feeling physically encumbered, weighted down), banksia robur (lethargy), cerato (strength to trust one's own judgment), larch (lack of self-confidence)
FOURTH: Heart	Bush fuchsia (speaking your true essence), crowea (worry), flannel flower (intimacy), sturt desert pea (emotional pain), holly (blocked love), gorse (despair)
FIFTH: Throat	Turkey bush (creative blocks)

SIXTH:

Third-eye (brow)   Bush iris (clears blocks relating to
                                 grounding and trust), bush fuscia
                                 (promotes intuition), isopogon
                                 (supports memory)

SEVENTH:

Crown   Red lily (disconnection), sundew
                                 (indecision), wild oat (reconnect-
                                 ing)

- CREAM/LOTION: If what you need is just for now, put
  some cream in your hand, add the required stock essence
  drops and mix before applying. To prepare a flower essence
  cream (think stretch marks for example), fill a glass jar with
  50g cream (you can use your favourite moisturizer as a base,
  but avoid any strongly scented creams). Add four drops of
  each chosen flower essence (up to four flower essences at a
  time). Mix with a wooden stick or stiff drinking straw. One
  or two drops of an essential oil can be added to the cream to
  enhance its healing properties. Apply to the area twice daily,
  or as required.
- HEALING: Put the remedy on your hands before doing
  energy work such as Reiki, Wiccan, or shamanic practices on
  yourself.
- MASSAGE: Mixing essences in massage oil can greatly enhance your mood. Put four drops of essential oil, one or two
  drops of relevant flower essence, and 50ml of jojoba oil into a
  glass bottle. Mix and use immediately. Recommended oils for
  this are: rose, ylang ylang, neroli or lavender. Ask someone to
  massage your lower back (another one to remember during
  birthing).

- TO ENHANCE BODYWORK: Flower essences are powerful tools when used in conjunction with acupuncture, energy work, massage, craniosacral therapy (this therapy is excellent for the newborn as it helps to heal birth trauma), or chiropractic treatments. Taking a few drops of flower essences before, during, and/or after a treatment helps the body "hold" positive adjustments by assisting the nervous system with repatterning as well as releasing the emotional/mental blocks.
- SUBTLE ENERGY MASSAGE: Place a few drops of your chosen flower essence on your hands and give yourself a subtle energy massage.
  1. Keep your hands about two inches away from your body. Move your right hand from the heart area down the inside of your left arm and up the outside. Swap sides and do the same for the other arm.
  2. Move your hands over the heart area, up over the head to the neck, and round to under the chin. Move down to under the breast area, round to the back (kidney area), and down over the buttocks and the back of the legs, imagining the movement going under the feet.
  3. Return your hands to the heart area and move both hands down over the torso and down the front of both legs, imagining the movement going under the feet.
- ROOMS: You could put a flower essence mixture in a bowl of water on the mantelpiece or table, or add your chosen oils to your burner and drop in four drops of flower essence. Another idea is to make up a spray as in the instructions for creating a body spray above and use on bedding or in a room. **Tip:** You might like to do this one for baby's room.

JANE'S JOURNEY

I mainly used Australian Bush remedies to help with my racing mind and disturbed sleep. This has been an issue throughout my pregnancy. I've had increasingly vivid dreams, found it hard to get back to sleep, and have often woken with a tense jaw. The flower remedies have really helped to quieten my mind. The ones that Laurel suggested I use were: macrocarpa, bottlebrush, black-eyed susan, crowea, and wild potato bush.

What Happens Next?

While flower essences can contribute to improving our mindset, we can also develop the habit of relaxation and meditation as a useful mind-body skill. It can also enhance chakra healing, ritual, and quartz crystal healing. Curious? Turn the page, gentle reader.

Useful Resources

Healing Waters (suppliers of Australian Bush Flower Essences)
www.essencesonline.com

CHAPTER 6

Relaxation and Meditation

L earning to relax on a regular basis will not only calm your mind but will prepare your body for a positive birth experience. When we are in pain, as when we are birthing, we tend to tense our mind and body, which makes any discomfort worse. Learning to relax throughout your pregnancy will make relaxation easier during the birth process.

Learning to relax helps:
- increase the hormone melatonin, boosting immunity, improving sleep, and raising mood.
- lower blood pressure, lessening the risk of preeclampsia.
- produce endorphins, the hormone that reduces pain.
- increase dehydroepiandrosterone (DHEA), an adrenal hormone that supports the immune system and improves brain chemistry, which can prevent pre- and post-pregnancy depression.

You could record any of the following relaxations or visualizations to reuse or ask someone to talk you through them.

Progressive Muscular Relaxation (PMR)

One of the simplest and most easily learned techniques for relaxation is Progressive Muscle Relaxation (PMR), a procedure widely used today that was originally developed by American physician Edmund Jacobson in the 1920s. The PMR procedure teaches you to relax your muscles through a two-step process. First you deliberately apply tension to certain muscle groups to gain familiarity with how your muscles feel when tense. Then you stop the tension and turn your attention to noticing how the muscles relax. In order to successfully use PMR during the birthing process, practise the technique daily throughout your pregnancy and become familiar with using it for relaxation.

PMR Script

Find a comfortable place to sit, away from interruptions. Feel the chair supporting your body. Your feet are firmly on the floor, your hands rest lightly on your thighs. Take in a deep breath and exhale completely.

- Bring your awareness down to your right foot. Curl your toes under your right foot as tight as you can. Hold the foot tight and feel the tension. Let the toes go. Feel the relaxation in the muscles in your feet and toes.
- Now curl your toes under on your left foot as tight as you can. Hold them tight and feel the tension. Let the toes go. Feel the relaxation in your feet and toes.
- Tighten the muscles in your right foot by splaying your foot out. Hold it tight. Feel the tension. Let the foot go. Feel the relaxation in the muscles in your foot and toes.
- Now tighten the muscles in your left foot by splaying your foot out. Hold it tight and feel the tension. Let the foot go. Feel the relaxation in the muscles in your foot and toes.
- Take a deep breath and exhale it completely.
- Tighten the front of the right leg by pointing your foot away from you so that it is almost parallel with your leg. Hold the right leg tight and feel the tension. Now let the foot go. Feel the relaxation in the muscles in your leg, foot, and toes.
- Now tighten the front of the left leg by pointing your foot away from you so that it is almost parallel with your leg. Hold the left

leg tight and feel the tension. Now let the foot go. Feel the relaxation in the muscles in your leg, foot, and toes.

- Tighten the back of the right leg by flexing your foot upwards, stretching from your heel down. Hold the right leg tight and feel the tension. Now let the foot go. Feel the relaxation in the muscles in your leg, foot, and toes.
- Now tighten the back of the left leg by flexing your foot upwards, stretching from your heel down. Hold the left leg tight and feel the tension. Now let the foot go. Feel the relaxation in the muscles in your leg, foot, and toes.
- Breathe deeply, exhale completely.
- Tighten the muscles in your right thigh while pressing your knee down into the floor. Hold them tight. Now let them go. Feel the relaxation in the muscles in your right thigh. Feel the relaxation in your calves, feet, and toes.
- Now tighten all the muscles in your left thigh while pressing your knee down into the floor. Hold them tight. Now let them go. Feel the relaxation in the muscles in your left thigh. Feel the relaxation in the muscles in your calves, feet, and toes.
- Keep breathing. We often hold a breath when we have tension in the body. Inhale deeply and exhale completely.
- Tighten the muscles in your buttocks by clenching your buttocks together. Hold them tight. Now let them go. Feel the relaxation in the muscles in your buttocks and thighs. Feel the relaxation in the muscles in your calves, feet, and toes.
- Tighten the muscles in your stomach by drawing in your stomach. Hold them tight. Now relax them. Let them go. Feel the relaxation in the muscles in your stomach and your buttocks. Feel the relaxation in the muscles in your thighs. Feel the relaxation in the muscles in your calves, feet, and toes.
- You're breathing deeply and easily.

- Tighten the muscles in your chest by breathing in. Hold your breath, and tighten all your chest muscles. Hold them tight. Now let them go. Feel the relaxation in the muscles in your chest and stomach. Feel the relaxation in the muscles in your buttocks and thighs. Feel the relaxation in the muscles in your calves, feet, and toes.
- Take in a deep breath and exhale completely, feeling even more relaxed.
- Tighten the muscles in your shoulders by pulling them up and forward. Hold them tight. Now let them go. Feel the relaxation in the muscles in your shoulders, chest, and stomach. Feel the relaxation in the muscles in your buttocks and thighs. Feel the relaxation in the muscles in your calves, feet, and toes.
- Now tighten the muscles in your shoulders by pulling them back. Hold them tight. Now let them go. Feel the relaxation in the muscles in your shoulders, chest, and stomach. Feel the relaxation in the muscles in your buttocks and thighs. Feel the relaxation in the muscles in your calves, feet, and toes.
- Breathe deeply and exhale completely.
- Tighten the muscles in your right hand, making it into a fist. Hold it tightly. Now let the hand go. Feel the relaxation in the muscles in your right hand and shoulders. Feel the relaxation in the muscles in your chest and stomach. Feel the relaxation in your buttocks and thighs. Feel the relaxation in your calves, feet, and toes.
- Now tighten the muscles in your left hand, making it into a fist. Hold it tightly. Now let the hand go. Feel the relaxation in the muscles in your left hand and shoulders. Feel the relaxation in the muscles in your chest and stomach. Feel the

relaxation in your buttocks and thighs. Feel the relaxation in your calves, feet, and toes.

- Take in a relaxing breath and exhale completely.
- Tighten the muscles in your right arm by tightening the biceps and lower arm together, but without the hand. Hold it tight. Now let it go. Feel the relaxation in your right arm, hand, and shoulders. Feel the relaxation in your chest and stomach. Feel the relaxation in your buttocks and thighs. Feel the relaxation in your calves, feet, and toes.
- Now tighten the muscles in your left arm by tightening the biceps and lower arm together, but without the hand. Hold it tight. Now let it go. Feel the relaxation in your left arm, hand, and shoulders. Feel the relaxation in your chest and stomach. Feel the relaxation in your buttocks and thighs. Feel the relaxation in your calves, feet, and toes. Feel yourself becoming more and more relaxed.
- Breathe deeply. Exhale completely.
- Now for a second time, tighten the muscles in your shoulders by pulling them up and forward or back. Hold them tight. Now let them go. Feel the relaxation in the muscles in your shoulders, arms, and hands. Feel the relaxation in your chest and stomach. Feel the relaxation in your buttocks and thighs. Feel the relaxation in your calves, feet, and toes.
- Breathing deeply and easily.
- Now tighten all the muscles in your neck. Stretch your head up, as if your chin could touch the ceiling. Then bend your head forward until your chin reaches your chest. Hold them very tight. Now soften all the muscles in your neck, shoulders, arms, and hands. Feel the relaxation in your chest and stomach. Feel the relaxation in your buttocks and thighs. Feel the relaxation in your calves, feet, and toes.

- Breathing deeply and easily.
- Now, tighten the muscles around your mouth and jaw by pressing your lips together and clenching your teeth. Hold them tight. Now release them. Feel the relaxation in the muscles in your mouth and jaw, your neck, shoulders, arms, and hands. Feel the relaxation in your chest and stomach. Feel the relaxation in your buttocks and thighs. Feel the relaxation in your calves, feet, and toes.
- Now tighten the muscles in your forehead and scalp by raising your eyebrows as if they could disappear. Hold them tightly. Now let them go. Feel the relaxation in the muscles around your mouth and jaw, your neck, shoulders, arms, and hands. Feel the relaxation in your chest and stomach. Feel the relaxation in your buttocks and thighs. Feel the relaxation in your calves, feet, and toes.
- Now tighten the muscles in your face by screwing all the muscles up together. Hold them tightly. Now let them go. Feel the relaxation in the muscles in your face, around your mouth and jaw. Feel the relaxation in the muscles in your neck, shoulders, arms, and hands. Feel the relaxation in your chest. Feel the relaxation in your stomach. Feel the relaxation in your buttocks and thighs. Feel the relaxation in your calves, feet, and toes.
- Breathe in deeply and exhale completely.
- Now allow your mind to slowly scan your body from your head to toes, to be certain that there's no tension lingering in any muscles anywhere. And if you find any tension, focus your mind on relaxing that remaining part of you completely. You feel completely relaxed from head to toe. You are more relaxed than you have been in a long while. Enjoy this time of deep relaxation. When you feel ready, open your eyes.

WISE WOMAN WAYS

Journaling your way through pregnancy can be incredibly helpful. I've used journaling throughout my adult life: when I had breast cancer, through relationship difficulties, family issues, and a work crisis. All you need is paper and pen. Your command of the language doesn't matter—only your intent to externalize your thoughts and feelings. No one else need read your words or gaze on your doodling. Journaling has helped me work through problems and externalize difficult personal thoughts I wouldn't dream of telling anyone.

Create Your Special Place For Baby Bonding

The purpose of this visualization is to help you imagine in your mind's eye a special place where you feel safe, comfortable, and relaxed with your baby, so that you can have time and space to bond. This place might be somewhere you know well or somewhere you create.

Close your eyes and take several slow, deep breaths. Now imagine a place where you feel completely safe, comfortable, and peaceful. It might be real or imaginary. Allow your special place to take shape visually through colours, textures, and shapes. Listen to the sounds of your special place; water, music, animals, or the sounds of nature. You may feel a light wind touch your face or warm sun soothing your skin. You may feel grass between your toes, soft sand beneath your feet, or the support of a comfortable chair. Pick up a favourite object from your special place and use your fingertips to explore it. Take a deep breath and notice all the rich fragrances around you—the scent of a flower, the tang of sea air, or the aroma of a special food you enjoy. Relax into the serenity, comfort, and safety of the special place you share with your baby.

Breathing easily and deeply. As you inhale, visualize your breath going down to your belly and baby.

Visualize a white or pink light surrounding you and your baby. This light is protecting and nourishing you both. Every part of your mind and body is filled with this powerful light. Feel it move deeper and deeper into every cell and organ of you and your baby, cleansing, opening, and balancing you both. You and your baby are completely safe and loved. Your mind becomes calm and clear and a sense of renewed peace and strength fills you. Say to yourself: "My baby and I are safe. My baby and I are well. My baby and I are loved. As I move through this pregnancy, my power as a woman and as a mother-to-be grows ever more powerful."

You feel peaceful and easy in your special place—a place that is always here. Take this time to talk to your baby, speak to him or her with kind, gentle, and loving words about the journey you share together. You know this mindset is a place you can visit anytime; it is a place where you can experience this healing energy and bond with your baby in peace.

When you are ready to return, take a deep breath and exhale fully. Open your eyes and spend a few moments enjoying this relaxed and comfortable feeling with your baby.

WISE WOMAN WAYS

The Adi Shakti mantra connects us to the Divine Mother. It is said that chanting this mantra eliminates fears and fulfills desires:

- I bow to (or call on) the primal power.
- I bow to (or call on) the all-encompassing power and energy.
- I bow to (or call on) that through which God creates.
- I bow to (or call on) the creative power of the Kundalini, the Divine Mother Power.

Relaxation Through Better Breathing

When stressed, breathing becomes shallow. There are two ways of breathing: chest or abdominal (belly). Chest breathing is shallow, irregular, and fast, and the body does not receive the correct amount of oxygen. A tipoff to this is that a person will continually sigh as a means of getting extra oxygen into the system, which provides short-term relief. This type of pattern often causes a person to hold their breath, hyperventilate, and experience shortness of breath. On top of this, the stress response will be activated, increasing anxiety and shallow breathing still further. This type of breathing is also associated with mouth breathing, which the body immediately associates with stress. Breathing through the nose automatically soothes the system and leads to fuller belly breathing.

The other main way of breathing is abdominal, or belly, breathing. Belly breathing is the way we are supposed to breathe and a sign of health. Just watch a newborn baby breathing and you will see; it is adults who forget how to do this. On inhaling through the nose, the lungs open fully to allow as much oxygen to enter the system as possible. The diaphragm contracts and expands to allow the lungs to expand, which naturally causes the belly to push out. This means the body has the right levels of oxygen to provide energy.

Abdominal breathing

Abdominal breathing can be very soothing because it slows you down. It is also efficient, bringing a good supply of oxygen to your brain. Check your breathing pattern by putting one hand on your chest and one hand on your stomach. If your lower hand moves and your top hand does not, you are doing abdominal breathing. But if your top hand moves and your bottom one does not, you are doing chest breathing.

You're going to inhale through your nose and exhale out of your mouth. Your exhalation needs to be longer than your inhalation. To slow your exhalation down, let your breath gently out, just enough to flicker a candle (purse your lips).

- Lay down flat and place your hands fingertip to fingertip, with your middle fingers meeting at your belly button, the palms of your hands lightly resting on your body.
- As you inhale through your nose, push your belly up and feel your fingertips expand. Rest a beat before exhaling slowly through your mouth. Rest a beat before inhaling again and feel your belly rise. Repeat this cycle five times.
- Now place your hands under the breast area of each side of your body, which is the rib area.
- As you inhale through your nose, expand your ribs and feel your hands push out. Rest a beat before exhaling slowly through your mouth. Feel your hands moving in again. Rest a beat before inhaling again and feel your ribs expand. Repeat this cycle five times.
- Now you are going to do a complete breathing cycle, inhaling deeply from the belly and ribcage and then exhaling completely.
- As you inhale through your nose for a count of five, push your belly up and expand your ribs. Rest a beat before exhaling slowly through your mouth for a count of six. Rest a beat before inhaling again and feel your belly rise and your ribs expand. Repeat this cycle five times.

The more you practise abdominal breathing, the easier it will become. Eventually, you will be able to do it anywhere—sitting, standing, or lying down.

WISE WOMAN WAYS

Incredibly easy ways to chill:

- Going for a walk with no aim in mind, nothing to do and no money on you to buy anything (apart from maybe a cup of something good!)
- Tuck yourself up in a quiet and comfortable place and go to sleep in the middle of the day.
- Indulge in a spell of comfort food, such as mashed potato, tomato soup, hot chocolate... well, you know the kind of thing.
- Buy something you have always wanted, can afford, and is a total waste of time and money—but it makes you incredibly happy.
- Sing lullabies to your baby.
- Lay in the grass watching the clouds through sleepy eyes.
- Lay on the beach with closed eyes, listening to the surf and the muted sounds of people around you.
- Lay under a tree.
- Paddle along the seashore's edge—as far as you can, as long as you like.
- Take a long walk by a long river.

Body Scan

Sit or lay down in a comfortable place where you won't be disturbed and close your eyes. Take a slow, deep breath through your nose and exhale completely. And again. Allow your body to become comfortable as you breathe deeply and easily.

Focus your awareness on your forehead and scalp. Allow any tension in the forehead and scalp to drain over the back of the head and out of the base of your neck into infinity. You're breathing easily and deeply. Releasing and relaxing. Your eyes are gently closed. Ease away the frown. Wiggle your jaw from side to side to loosen the tension. Your tongue should be behind your lower teeth. You're breathing easily and deeply.

- Focus your awareness on your right shoulder and arm. Allow any tension in the right shoulder and arm to drain down the arm. Down, down, down the arm, out the fingers, and into infinity.
- Focus your awareness on your left shoulder and arm. Allow any tension in the left shoulder and arm to drain down the arm. Down, down, down the arm, out the fingers, and into infinity. You're breathing easily and deeply. Releasing and relaxing.
- Focus on the chest area. Feel the chest area opening and expanding. You're breathing easily and deeply.
- Focus on the stomach. Allow the stomach to relax. Releasing and relaxing.
- Focus your awareness on the back area. Upper back, middle back, and lower back. Allow any tension in the back area to slide down the spine. Down, down, down the spine, out the base of the spine, into infinity. You're breathing easily and deeply. Releasing and relaxing.
- Focus your attention on your right hip and leg. Allow any tension in the right hip and leg to drain down the leg. Down, down, down the leg, out the toes, into infinity.
- Focus your attention on your left hip and leg. Allow any tension in the left hip and leg to drain down the leg. Down, down, down the leg, out the toes, into infinity. Releasing and relaxing.
- You feel completely relaxed from head to toe—more relaxed than you have been in a long while.

JANE'S JOURNEY

Towards the end of my pregnancy Laurel invited me to a half-day workshop where I could explore some relaxation and meditation techniques around natural pain management. We tailored these to fit in with what felt right for me and what fitted in with some of the practices I had already learned at my pregnancy yoga classes. A benefit of having reflexology with Laurel was that I could learn to apply my pain management techniques during the more "uncomfortable" reflexology moments!

What Happens Next?

Now that you're blissed out, you might feel inclined to make love. Did you know that sex resets your nervous system and can naturally trigger the relaxation response? When your mind and hormones are in the mood, you can enjoy sex throughout your pregnancy. Aroused enough to turn the page?

CHAPTER 7

Sex and Pregnancy

You can't harm your baby by making love, so enjoy! The cervix is protected from infection by a thick mucus plug, while the muscles of your womb and the cushion of the amniotic sac keep your baby safe.

Caution!

If you have a history of abdominal pain, bleeding, miscarriage, premature birthing; if your partner has genital herpes; if you have cervical weakness, cramps, or a low-lying placenta; talk with your midwife, doula, or doctor before making love.

> **WISE WOMAN WAYS**
> Nausea should lift during the second trimester, boosting estrogen levels and improving your sex drive. Most studies show that this trimester is the time when women feel the most sexual desire.

Let's Talk Positions

As your pregnancy progresses, you will probably need to find different positions for penetrative sex. Here's a few to get your creative juices going:

- Lie on your sides facing each other. Pull up one leg to allow room for your partner. This position might be more pleasant in the first two trimesters.

- Woman on top (he lies face up and you straddle him, facing him or the feet) can give great levels of sexual satisfaction during pregnancy. It puts no weight on your abdomen and allows you to control the depth of penetration. This position is also called the cowgirl position or when facing the feet, reverse cowgirl.
- Lying side by side in the spoons position, with your man behind you, allows for shallow penetration from the rear and is great for the last few months of pregnancy.
- Woman lying down (best in first trimester). Lie on your back with a pillow under your bottom for support and raise your knees up towards your chest with your partner kneeling between your legs.
- The doggy position is good for later on in pregnancy. Get on all fours, using pillows to support your stomach and chest. To prevent deep penetration, ask your partner to put a pillow or cushion between his tummy and your bottom.
- Making love sitting down is another position that puts no weight on your womb. Sit on your partner's lap (facing him or not, as you like) as he sits on a chair. You can control the rate and depth of penetration by squatting or standing up more.

> **WISE WOMAN WAYS**
> You may find that you can experience more pleasure from masturbation than intercourse. Masturbation is a great release of sexual energy and is great if you're not interested in penetration or if only one of you is interested in sex at that moment.

Let's Talk Orgasms

In general, orgasms are very good for you and baby! When you have an orgasm, the baby is unaware of what you are doing but does experience the euphoric hormone rush that you experience.

Many women find that their clitoris is slightly less sensitive during pregnancy or that their orgasms are less powerful. Other women may experience their first orgasm during pregnancy due to the clitoris and vagina becoming more sensitive due to increased fluids in the area.

If you orgasm, you may notice your baby moves around more because of your pounding heart—not because baby knows what's happening or feels discomfort.

You may find orgasms make your bump change shape as the muscles contract squeezing the baby gently (baby is quite safe).

On my research travels for this chapter I happily came across "orgasmic meditation," or "OMing" (a term coined by Nicole Daedone), which is a mindfulness practice where the focus of meditation is conscious finger to genital contact. Your partner gently holds your genitals and precisely and slowly strokes your clitoris using his index finger for 15 minutes. Both of you place your complete awareness mindfully on that localized point of contact between you, focusing your full attention on your sensitive nerve endings, to develop connective resonance between you both. The outcome is orgasm and intimate personal connection with your partner.

> **WISE WOMAN WAYS**
>
> In the third trimester, an orgasm can set off surges. If this happens, you'll feel the muscles of your womb go hard. This is perfectly normal. If it feels uncomfortable, do your relaxation techniques or lie quietly until the surges pass.

Keep Talking

The most important piece of advice I can give you is to encourage the communication between you. This is a time of profound change for you both. Your relationship and lifestyle is changing and will continue to do so after the birth. Even though you are the one carrying a child, there are three of you already.

If you feel positive about your pregnancy, you're likely to feel more sexual. But if you're not particularly happy about the pregnancy, or feel insecure about other issues, such as the relationship, this can have a negative effect on your sexual relationship.

Think of where your partner may be coming from. Common reasons for lack of desire in dads-to-be include:

- fears that sex can hurt the baby
- thinking of you as a mother, therefore not associating you with sex
- worries about you and your unborn baby's health
- feelings of apprehension about the burdens of parenthood
- self-consciousness about making love in the presence of your unborn child
- feeling edged out due to increased numbers of women around you

Your baby was created by the two of you, yet for the next nine months it is you who surrounds and carries the unborn child, while your partner is on the outside looking in. This is a sacred time for the two of you, as well as the three of you. In every relationship, there are three energies: you, your partner, and the dynamics you each bring to the third component: the relationship. The duality here is the inclusion of baby. Be mindful of nourishing the intimacy, including sexuality, of the relationship between you and your partner. Keep talking and sharing yourselves with each other. It is this intimacy that weaves into the bedrock of your relationship and on which your baby is carried.

WISE WOMAN WAYS

If sperm comes in contact with the neck of your womb when you are near or past your due date, it can help to trigger birthing by ripening the cervix and causing it to open up. This is because sperm contains a substance called prostaglandins (the same chemical that is used to induce birthing artificially).

What Happens Next?

Sexual expression can be made all the more sacred and fulfilling if you bring chakra healing into the weave. Read on to find out more.

CHAPTER 8

Chakra Healing

Think of yourself as an eclectic energy field of mind, body, and spirit—mind, with its intellect and emotions; the physical body; and the elusive spirit. Spiritual energy is less tangible, yet it permeates and underpins all the other energy fields. In addition to healing the mind and body during pregnancy, we need to look at nourishing the energetic body that is part of our spiritual nature.

To grasp spiritual energy, we need to have some concept of the Divine or the sacred. These two words could be defined as the infinite, the everlasting, God, Goddess, or universal energy. We may reflect that our human connection to the sacred is through our sense of spirituality, like an umbilical cord. You and your baby, separately and together, have that link to the sacred.

Our awareness of our spirituality, our connection to the Divine, develops throughout our lifetime (or several). Metaphorically, you might consider your spirituality as a flame deep within you that burns brighter as you become more conscious.

WISE WOMAN WAYS

When I teach students about energetic anatomy, I explain it this way. Imagine you are a ball of light. This is your eternal flame, your link with the sacred, your spiritual self. In order for its brightness and connectedness to grow, you need to become increasingly aware of the defenses it has around it that dim its glow—defenses such as ego, anger, fear, and so on.

As you become more aware of yourself and work to let go of the mindsets that hold you back, more of these defenses will begin to fall away, allowing the ball of light to burn brighter still, increasing your connectedness to the sacred.

Imagine covering this ball of light in something like a loose-weave cloth. You can see the cloth, but because the weave is so loose, you can also see the glow of the ball through the cloth. This cloth represents your energy anatomy: your auric field and your chakra system. Energetic anatomy isn't a physical thing; it's a subtle energy manifestation and is as important as your physical anatomy. The energy field is like a multi-gateway system, through which you give and receive mental, emotional, physical, and spiritual energy. The more your ball glows and grows, the more the weave of your energy field expands. The development of your energetic anatomy and your ball of light become increasingly one and the same.

The chakra system is part of your energy anatomy system and consists of several major chakras and many minor chakras. The word *chakra* is a Sanskrit word, meaning "vortex" or "wheel." These chakras aren't on the physical body but on the etheric body (part of your auric energy field). A major chakra resembles a spinning wheel. When balanced, it spins appropriately. If the chakra is blocked, the spin may be slower, counter-clockwise, or static. When overstimulated, the chakra may be spinning too fast.

Each chakra has a relationship to our physical body as well as to psychological mindsets. Our chakra system evolves as we grow older. This chapter will help you engage with chakra healing, as you travel through pregnancy.

The Chakra System

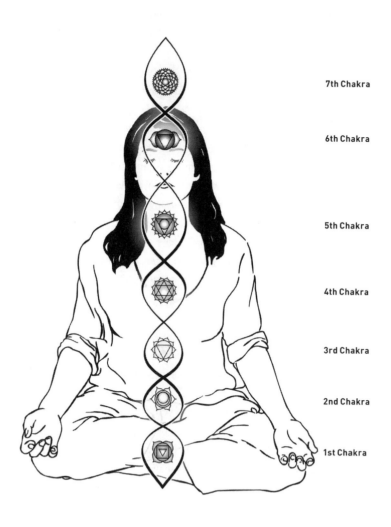

7th Chakra

6th Chakra

5th Chakra

4th Chakra

3rd Chakra

2nd Chakra

1st Chakra

Grounding Yourself

Before starting to perform any type of chakra healing, it is important to ground yourself. Grounding allows you to remain firmly connected to the earth by perceiving yourself anchored by roots that extend down to the core of the earth via your root chakra, for example. It prevents you from feeling "floaty" or "spaced out."

A grounding exercise

Sit or stand with eyes closed and observe your breathing for a few minutes. Visualize yourself as a tree, with roots growing down into the earth through the soles of your feet. The energy of your being roots deep into the earth and any excess energy is grounded within your strong roots. When you feel you are sufficiently anchored or earthed, bring yourself back into the room.

Other grounding techniques include: abdominal, or belly, breathing; physical exercise; eating something; being in nature; and putting your hands into sand, soil, or running water.

> **WISE WOMAN WAYS**
> Just as you have a sacred connection to the Divine, so your baby has a sacred connection to the Divine as well. During these nine months, you and baby are joined, each with the other, in Divinity.

Protecting Yourself And Your Baby

Whenever we are consciously working with our chakras, we open ourselves up to receiving the universal healing energy and are more sensitive to the energies around us. To protect against draining energies, there are a number of techniques you can use.

A protection exercise

Wrap a protective cloak of light and vitality around yourself and your baby, covering from head to toe. Visualize it as any colour that offers strength, comfort, and reassurance (blue is good). Request that universal energy, God, or Goddess protect you both from all negative energy.

Cleansing Yourself

Our chakras need cleansing regularly to get rid of unwanted energies absorbed from people, places, or situations. If you are feeling tired, drained, or emotionally unstable, you may be absorbing and carrying external energies and this may have an influence on you and baby. Daily cleansing will help to clear these energies and improve the circulation of your own energies, thereby improving the energy to you both.

It is also important to make sure that you have carried out a cleansing exercise before you perform self-healing practices for yourself or your unborn child. The clearer your chakras and aura are, the more healing energy you will be able to create, attract, and absorb.

A cleansing exercise

First ground and protect yourself and your baby. Smudge sticks are a traditional way of cleansing, using a bound stick of sage and sweetgrass. Light the smudge stick and wave it around your body to cleanse your physical body, your aura, and chakras. If you have asthma or allergies, you might like to use a flower essence spray instead.

Now start to get a sense of your auric energy field. Feel how far it extends into the space around you. See and sense its layers with your inner vision. Ask the Divine to remove all negative energy within your energy field immediately and to send it instantly to the Light. Ask the Divine to cleanse, heal, and protect your energy field for the highest good of you and your baby. Once this cleansing exercise is complete, bring your focus back to your breathing and your physical body.

WISE WOMAN WAYS

All this grounding, protecting, and cleansing can sound a tad woolly; however, an awareness of your subtle energy and a willingness to engage with it in a practical way will help you feel calmer and more positive. I can't guarantee that, of course! Try it and see for yourself.

Using Healing For Yourself And Baby

To engage with chakra healing is simple. Find a quiet place, free from distraction for you and baby. You may be sitting or lying down. Your eyes may be open or closed. Closed might encourage you to focus on your inner experience more. Take a few deep, slow breaths and relax your body as much as possible. Ground yourself and set your protection. Place your hand on the chakra and feel the warmth of your touch. Breathe into the place where your hand is—in and out, slowly and deeply. As you inhale, imagine breathing in peaceful, healing energy; as you exhale, imagine this same energy flowing out of your hand and into the chakra.

Cautions!

This next section gives an overview of the seven major chakras and how you might work with each chakra during your pregnancy, including yoga positions. Consult a qualified pregnancy yoga teacher, as you may need more advice before trying these positions, depending on where you are in your pregnancy. For more information see *The Yoga of Pregnancy* by Mel Campbell (see page 159).

While there are several aromatherapy oils you can use to improve the well-being of yourself and your baby, if you have any doubts or concerns about which oils are safe to use, consult a qualified aromatherapist.

Working With the Chakras
During the Pregnancy

CHAKRA	1
Yin and Yang poles	Yin (receptive and feminine)
Location	Base of spine between anus and genitals at the perineum, connected to coccyx and opening downwards
Sensory function	Smell
Associated body parts	Skeletal system, adrenal glands, kidneys, anus, prostate, bladder, and genitals
Physical dysfunction	Osteoporosis and adrenal fatigue
Pregnancy/birthing issues	Imbalance may result in early or quick birthing, inability to open cervix, resulting in long birthing or caesarean
Life issues	Survival, physical needs, standing up for oneself, physical health and fitness, grounding, stability, security, group power, and identity
Emotional dysfunction	Mental lethargy, "spaciness," victim mentality, unfocused mind, and distrust
Behaviourial dysfunction	Difficulty achieving goals, overactivity, passivity, not looking after one's body
Colour	Red/black
Element	Earth
Australian Bush Essences	Waratah, red lily (disconnection), sundew (indecisive), fringe violet (aura damage), grey spider (panic),

	macrocarpa (exhaustion), and bush iris (clearing blocks of physical excess and materialism)
Bach Flower Remedies	Rock rose (extreme panic and fears), clematis (daydreamer, too much time in the spirit realm, ungrounded), hornbeam (mental exhaustion), aspen (vague fears of the unknown)
Aromatherapy oils	Sandalwood, patchouli, musk
Quartz crystals	Red tiger's eye, garnet, red jasper, ruby, obsidian, hematite, agate, bloodstone, garnet, red coral, ruby, hematite, onyx, rose quartz, smoky quartz
Yoga positions	Bridge (with progressing pregnancy) *– advisable to practice with bolster/ block under the sacrum;* Balancing *– with progressing pregnancy: advisable to use a wall as support* Child pose, Spinal roll, Half and full locust *– avoid if experiencing SPD (Symphysis Pubis Dysfunction) / PGD (Pelvic Girdle Discomfort)*

Reflections

- What are your physical needs during your pregnancy at this time?
- How is your identity changing now that you are a mother?
- To what extent are you integrating with other mums-to-be? How does your choice feel to you?

I recognize when this chakra is out because I can get lower back pain and constipation, while psychologically I know that I'm not trusting myself or another person about something. If you'll excuse the pun, this chakra for me can be a pain in the bum!

> **WISE WOMAN WAYS**
> The balance of your chakra system will have an effect on your baby, both during the pregnancy and on into the baby's life. So the more thoughtful and proactive you are in your chakra healing, the better it will be for both of you.

CHAKRA	2 (this is obviously a sensitive chakra during pregnancy and I would recommend that you avoid direct healing on this centre during this time)
Yin and Yang poles	Yang (positive and masculine)
Location	Lower abdomen, between naval and genitals, just above the anus, opens forward
Sensory function	Taste
Associated body parts	Circulatory system, uterus, ovaries, and testes glands
Physical dysfunction	Impotence, frigidity, bladder and prostate trouble, lower back pain, and erratic libido
Pregnancy/birthing issues	This chakra is incredibly influenced by baby, which may result in you experiencing intuitive dreams

Life issues	Emotional balance, sexuality, uncovering motivations, influencing choices based on conditioning, allowing pleasure, creative expression, partnerships, and playfulness
Emotional dysfunction	Instability, sadness, feelings of isolation, and martyr mentality
Behaviourial dysfunction	Excessive libido, sexual withdrawal
Colour	Orange
Element	Water
Australian Bush Essences	Turkey bush (creativity), billy goat plum (releases shame), spinifex (cleansing, victim archetype), she oak (hormonal imbalance), and flannel flower (lack of sensitivity, especially in males, and sexual abuse)
Bach Flower Remedies	Agrimony, centaury, pine, larch, and gorse
Aromatherapy oils	Melissa, orange, mandarin, neroli, sandalwood and ylang ylang
Quartz crystals	Coral, carnelian, citrine, and golden topaz
Yoga positions	Pelvic rock, Goddess pose, Pelvic side rolls, Open legs, Downward facing dog
	– *avoid in the later stage of the third trimester*
	Cobra
	– *avoid after the first trimester*
	Hip circles (see Chakra 1)
	– *avoid if experiencing SPD or PGD*

Reflections

- What influences might you be carrying from your past that influence your thoughts now as a mother?
- How has your dream life changed since you have become pregnant?
- How are you allowing pleasure to enter your life as you go through pregnancy?

Ah, the chakra of creative self-expression. At the time of writing this book—when my uterus has a fluid life of its own—my creative side is struggling to be birthed on a more profound level. I've never birthed a physical baby, but by jingo, birthing the baby of creativity surely comes a close second!

The womb is occupied by a growing baby developing its own system of chakras. Your sacral chakra becomes the sacred seat of the baby's soul.

The lesson of the sacral chakra is letting go of fear, anger, and controlling behaviour so that the purpose of the Sacred is achieved through emotional connections to the baby growing inside of you and to the Divine Mother within. Letting go of past limitations so that the creativity of your new life can flourish. Letting go of the fear of the unknown. Is my baby okay? Will I have a painful birth? Will I have enough milk? Will I have enough money?

The ultimate manifestation of the lesson of the sacral chakra is letting go in birthing and releasing inhibitions to trust that birth is for the sacred purpose of bonding with your baby. This bonding stimulates the baby's sacral chakra, and the emotional connection created between mother and child fulfills its sacred purpose and brings the sacral chakra into balance.

WISE WOMAN WAYS

I've often seen sparkle in a pregnant woman's energy field, which becomes like fine silver rain the nearer she gets to birthing.

CHAKRA	3
Yin and Yang poles	Yin (receptive and feminine)
Location	Between navel and base of sternum (solar plexus), opens forward
Sensory function	Sight
Associated body parts	Digestive system, gallbladder, spleen, pancreas, liver, limbic system, and adrenal glands
Physical dysfunction	Stomach ulcers, fatigue, weight around stomach, allergies, and diabetes
Pregnancy/birthing issues	Imbalance of this chakra can lead to pregnancy symptoms such as nausea, diabetes, and raised body temperature
Life issues	Personal power, will, self-esteem/ self-confidence, the courage to take risks, to be, purpose, effectiveness, endurance, self-respect, uniqueness, and individuality
Emotional dysfunction	Oversensitive to criticism, low self-esteem
Behaviourial dysfunction	Aggressive, controlling, addictions
Colour	Yellow
Element	Fire

Australian Bush Essences	Dynamis essence (combination of essences for energy), old man banksia (counteracts weariness), macrocarpa (energy), crowea (releases worry), wild potato bush (releases feeling physically encumbered, weighted down), banksia robur (lethargy), bottlebrush (bonding between mother and child, letting go), peach-flowered tea tree (mood swings), five corners (low self-confidence)
Bach Flower Remedies	Cerato (strength to trust one's own judgement), larch (lack of self-confidence), schleranthus (indecisiveness), pine (guilt)
Aromatherapy oils	Rosemary, lemon, grapefruit, bergamot, ginger, ylang ylang, and cinnamon
Quartz crystals	Citrine, amber, tiger's eye, yellow topaz
Yoga positions	Front Stretch, Belly push *– advisable to practice with knees bent* Warrior *– with progressing pregnancy: advisable to use a wall as support* Bow *– avoid after first trimester; can put too much strain and stretch to the abdominal muscles and uterus*

Reflections

- How is your self-esteem changing as you travel your journey through pregnancy?
- Are you taking on too much responsibility? Do you need to delegate?

> **WISE WOMAN WAYS**
> Continue to develop a conscious awareness of your energy anatomy. Sometimes I can be doing something inane and I become aware that my hand chakras are generating enormous heat. Waste not, want not—I channel this active healing energy to those in need.

CHAKRA	4
Yin and Yang poles	Yang (positive and masculine)
Location	Centre of chest (breastbone), opens forward
Sensory function	Feeling
Associated body parts	Heart, chest, lungs, circulation, and thymus gland
Physical dysfunction	Shallow breathing, high blood pressure, heart disease, and cancer
Pregnancy/birthing issues	You may find yourself experiencing difficult feelings about your ability to relate or share your love
Life issues	Beliefs about love and relationships, forgiveness and compassion for oneself and others, balance, compassion and self-acceptance, and unconditional acceptance of others

Emotional dysfunction	Co-dependency, melancholia, fears concerning loneliness, commitment, and/or betrayal
Behaviourial dysfunction	Passivity, withdrawal
Colour	Green/pink
Element	Air
Australian Bush Essences	Bush fuchsia (speaking your true essence), crowea (worry), turkey bush (creativity), red grevillia (becoming unstuck), flannel flower (intimacy), illawara flame tree (fear of rejection), sturt desert pea (emotional pain), bluebell, rough bluebell (disconnection from feeling)
Bach Flower Remedies	Holly (blocked love), gorse (despair), chicory
Aromatherapy oils	Eucalyptus, pine, tea tree, bergamot, and melissa
Quartz crystals	Aventurine, emerald, jade, malachite, peridot, rose quartz, watermelon tourmaline, green calcite, azurite, and moonstone
Yoga positions	Cow face, Cobra – *avoid after first trimester* Restorative reclined supported fish pose – *use block or support under back and head; otherwise too much strain along the front abdominal muscles and uterus*

> Breathing
> *– e.g. The golden circle breath from*
> *the heart centre to the baby and*
> *back to the heart centre*

Reflections

- How are your intimate relationships changing as a result of your pregnancy?
- Are there some issues you feel ready to forgive others (or yourself) for?

This heart chakra is, for me, maybe the most poignant of all. To experience self-love and self-respect is most challenging. Yet how can we truly love another or accept love from another, if we don't have this love and respect for the self?

CHAKRA	5
Yin and Yang poles	Yin (receptive and feminine)
Location	Centrally at base of neck, opens forward
Sensory function	Hearing
Associated body parts	Throat, ears, nose, teeth, mouth, neck, thyroid, and parathyroid glands
Physical dysfunction	Sore throats, neck ache, thyroid problems, hearing problems, tinnitus, and asthma
Pregnancy/birthing issues	This chakra assists you in protecting your baby from untoward influences from the outside world through intellect and rationality.

Life issues	Communication, self-expression, the power of choice, personal expression, harmony with others, self-knowledge, creativity
Emotional dysfunction	Perfectionism, inability to express emotions, and blocked creativity
Behaviourial dysfunction	Withdrawal, people pleasing
Colour	Light blue
Element	Sound
Australian Bush Essences	Cognis' essence (clarity and courage to speak truth, great for study and new information), paw paw (assimilating new information), turkey bush (creative blocks), old man banksia (weariness), bush fuchsia (imbalance of intuition and logic)
Bach Flower Remedies	Agrimony
Aromatherapy oils	Geranium or bergamot
Quartz crystals	Sodalite, lapis lazuli, blue agate, aquamarine, turquoise, celestite, sapphire
Yoga positions	Neck rolls, Restorative reclined supported fish pose
	– use block or support under back and head; otherwise too much strain along the front abdominal muscles and uterus
	Shoulder stand and Plough
	– advised to only practice in pregnancy when it was practiced prior to being pregnant

Reflections

- To what extent are you able to free yourself from harmful external values and beliefs?
- To what extent are you able to express yourself and your beliefs?
- To what extent might you be hiding yourself behind your pregnancy?

Many years ago, in my late twenties, I went through a particular growth phase when I was making connections with my "little Laurel" side and realizing how much of my inappropriate adult drives were happening because of unhealthy childhood conditioning. In one vision quest, I saw myself as a thin, naked little girl with a paper bag over her head. In the two weeks following this, I developed a cold and a horrendous cough, during which time (I hope this isn't too much information for you) phlegm caught in my throat by the bucketful necessitating an emergency visit by the doctor. My cough and cold came and went. More importantly, I learnt to express my feelings as an adult and to heal from past trauma.

CHAKRA	6
Yin and Yang poles	Yang (receptive and masculine)
Location	Above and between eyebrows, space behind forehead, opens forward
Sensory function	Sixth sense
Associated body parts	Eyes, base of skull, nose, ears, and pituitary gland
Physical dysfunction	Headaches, poor vision, neurological disturbances, glaucoma, and nightmares
Pregnancy/birthing issues	You will receive a boost to your intuition especially during birthing

Life issues	Intuition, wisdom, emotional intelligence, ability to "see" other than with the eyes
Emotional dysfunction	Seasonally depressed
Behaviourial dysfunction	Learning difficulties, hallucinations
Colour	Indigo
Element	Light
Australian Bush Essences	Bush iris (clears blocks relating to grounding and trust), bush fuchsia (intuition), isopogon (memory), green spider orchid, and boronia
Bach Flower Remedies	Walnut, crab apple, rock water, and vervain
Aromatherapy oils	Patchouli, frankincense, or bergamot
Quartz crystals	Tourmaline, tanzanite, lapis lazuli, sapphire, amethyst, purple apatite, azurite, calcite, and fluorite
Yoga positions	Palming, Seated yoga mudra, Visualization, Imagery

Reflections

- To what extent have your intuitive abilities sharpened during your pregnancy?
- How do you balance your imagination and fantasy realm with reality?
- To what extent do you hide your intuition behind a rational mind?

CHAKRA	7
Yin and Yang poles	Yin and Yang
Location	Top/crown of head, position of fontanels, opens upward
Sensory function	None
Associated body parts	Upper skull, cerebral cortex, skin, pineal gland
Physical dysfunction	Sensitivity to pollution, chronic exhaustion, epilepsy, and Alzheimer's disease
Pregnancy/birthing issues	This chakra brings the understanding that we are a temporary guardian to this baby and the first guide in its life
Life issues	Spirituality, selflessness, expanded consciousness
Emotional dysfunction	Depression, obsessive thinking, confusion
Behaviourial dysfunction	Obsessive-compulsive disorder (OCD)
Colour	Violet, white, and gold
Element	Thought, cosmic energy
Australian Bush Essences	Red lily (disconnection), sundew (indecision), angelsword (interference with spiritual connection) and bush iris (fear of death)
Bach Flower Remedies	Wild oat (reconnecting)
Aromatherapy oils	Frankincense
Quartz crystals	Amethyst, diamond, clear quartz, white jade, white tourmaline, snowy quartz, and herkimer.

Yoga positions   Hare Pose (Shashankasana),
Standing, Wide Angle Forward
Bend,
– possibly with head resting on block
Headstand
*– advised to only practice in preg-
nancy when it was practiced prior
to being pregnant*
Seated Meditation

Reflections

- To what extent do you experience your connection to the Divine, especially as your pregnancy develops?
- To what extent do you experience unconditional love in other intimate relationships?

> **WISE WOMAN WAYS**
>
> Do the following exercise, before going to bed at night or if you have been exposed to negative or scattered energy:
>
> 1   Using the third and fourth fingers of both hands, press firmly on the point between the eyebrows. From there, with the same fingers, trace a line over the crown of the head and down to the back of the neck and then down the spine as far as you can reach.
>
> 2   Still using the same fingers, reach under your arms and around to the centre of your back to pick up at the point you left off in step 1 and continue, pressing firmly down the centre of the back, the backs of the legs (simultaneously) to the calves. Finish with a flick of the fingers.

3   With the third and fourth fingers of the right hand, start again at the point between the eyebrows and trace a line up and over the crown, down the back of the neck, back under your right side of your chin, and along the left shoulder and the front of the left arm. Finish the movement with a sharp flick.

4   Repeat the steps above, this time using the third and fourth fingers of the left hand and tracing the line over the head and down the front of the right arm.

5   Using both hands, trace the line up from the point between the eyebrows over the head to the back of the neck. Here, the hands separate and go down each side of the neck under the jaw line, over the front of the throat, to join again at the breastbone. In one continuous flowing movement and maintaining firm pressure, follow the centre line down the front of the body with both hands and then (simultaneously) down both legs, finishing at the ankles, once again with a flick.

What Happens Next?

Chakra healing can deepen the relationship between you and your baby. Quartz crystal healing can further enhance this link. Let me tell you more.

CHAPTER 9

Using Quartz Crystals for Pregnancy

The composition of the earth is one-third quartz crystal and is one of the most abundant compounds found in the earth's surface and in most sedimentary, metamorphic, and igneous rocks. Quartz has also been found in lunar rocks. Did you know:

- the silica and water that crystals are composed of are also major components of the physical body?
- quartz is fossilized water, and our bodies are 65-75 percent water?
- crystals' piezoelectric effects (their energy fields) match the earth's magnetic field and the magnetic field of the human aura?

There is a huge variety of quartz and quartz derivatives, including the following: agate, amethyst, ametrine, aqua aura quartz, aventurine, black quartz, bloodstone, blue siberian quartz, candle quartz, carnelian, cathedral quartz, chalcedony, chrysoprase, citrine, clear quartz, drusy quartz, elestial quartz, faden quartz, fairy quartz, golden healer quartz, green siberian quartz, heliotrope, jasper, lavender quartz, lepidocrosite herkimer, metamorphosis quartz, onyx, opal, phantom quartz, rock crystal, rose quartz, ruby aura quartz, rutilated quartz, sardonyx, smoky quartz, snow quartz, spirit quartz, starseed quartz, quartz, tiger's eye, and tourmaline.

You can find quartz in many everyday items, including sandpaper, soap, ceramics, radios, and TVs. Quartz was the first crystal to be used in radio wave transceivers and is used in watches and timepieces; it was essential in the development of computers. When a crystal is put in a watch, the battery sends a constant charge through the crystal. The crystal absorbs the charge and then releases it at such a precise rate it is used to make the watch keep perfect time.

How Crystal Healing Works

The ancient Egyptians used lapis lazuli, turquoise, carnelian, emerald, and clear quartz in their jewellery and grave amulets. Stones were used for protection and health. A hieroglyphic papyrus from the year 2,000 BC documents a medical cure using crystal, and several from the year 1,500 BC have additional prescriptions.

Jade was seen as the concentrated essence of love and was recognized as a kidney healing stone both in China and South America.

The original settlers of North, Central, and South America used crystals widely for spiritual, ceremonial, and healing purposes. Mayan Indians used quartz crystals for both the diagnosis and treatment of disease.

In Europe, from the 11th century through the Renaissance, a number of medical treatises appeared (Hildegard von Bingen, Arnoldus Saxo, and John Mandeville), extolling the virtues of precious and semiprecious stones in the treatment of ailments, alongside herbal remedies.

The solar temple at Newgrange in the Boyne Valley of Ireland is older than the pyramids and was built so that the sun would stream through the 70-foot-long entrance tunnel on the Winter Solstice. Its roof was originally covered with white quartz, to symbolize the White Goddess.

Quartz crystals focus, structure, amplify, transmit, transform, and store energy because they:

- have an energy grid of their own that evolves;

- absorb the energy of the earth, nature, environment, events, and people around them and reveal their layers in response to different energies;
- have layers of growth and experience, as we do;
- and have their own karmic cycles.

American research scientist Marcel Vogel (1917–1991) worked for IBM for 27 years and developed the magnetic coating for IBM's disc drive and the first liquid crystal displays (LCD). He believed that the inner structure of crystals is in a perfect state of balance and radiates energy in a coherent manner that could be used to heal negative thought forms at the base of disease. Vogel also designed the Vogel Crystal, which focuses the universal life force.

Crystals affect the energy anatomy (chakras and aura) fields that surround and permeate the physical body. A quartz crystal may be held in the hand or placed around the body. The power of the crystal is directed to the part of the physical body or energetic anatomy that requires healing. Crystals complement other healing modalities. When placed on or around the body during a healing session and used in conjunction with other healing modalities, such as shamanic healing or Reiki, the crystals work both independently and cooperatively to create healing.

Crystals may be worn, placed in an environment (outside or inside), or even used in a distance healing capacity.

WISE WOMAN WAYS

I've always felt crystals, flowers, plants, herbs, and wood need to be placed together and try to do this aesthetically in the home as part of the décor.

Cleansing Crystals

Cleansing is the process of removing any previous energies and influences that a crystal may have absorbed or come into contact with, either during its production, handling, or environment of origin. It is a good idea to cleanse the crystals you work with on a regular basis.

Water

Place the crystal in a clear glass bowl filled with water. CAUTION: Some crystals are water-soluble, which means they can dissolve in water. Most water-soluble crystals end in "ite."

Salt

Most members of the quartz family are safe with salt, but some are not. Dissolve one teaspoon of sea salt in one pint of water and place your crystal in the water overnight. Make sure you rinse all traces of salt away from the crystal and allow the crystal to dry naturally. Or you can bury your crystal in a bowl of natural sea salt for eight hours. Make sure you brush away all remains of salt.

Smudging

You can smudge crystals with sage, myrrh, sandalwood, frankincense, lavender, cedar, thyme, rosemary, or sweetgrass to cleanse them. Either fan the incense over the crystals with a feather or pass the crystal through the smoke of burning herbs, incense, or essential oil several times.

Other crystals

You can cleanse your crystal by placing it on a large crystal cluster for several hours. Quartz clusters are self-cleaning and charging. Citrine is also a cleansing crystal in its own right.

Sunlight

You can cleanse your crystals by placing in direct sunlight (inside or outside), which is said to represent male energies. CAUTION: The sun will fade many crystals, including amethyst. Direct hot sun beaming through clear quartz may also be a fire hazard.

Moonlight

The moon can also cleanse crystals and is said to represent female energies. During the full moon, the moon's energy is enhanced and is a good time for cleaning crystals. Place the crystals outside or inside. CAUTION: Be aware of rain, if placing crystals outside. I've cleansed crystals this way many times and find it a wonderful experience. We have a very long, terraced garden, which slopes away from the house. Sometimes I've placed the crystals out at dusk, so I don't break my neck getting down the garden at night. I have placed extra protection around the crystal layout, and not once have I found any crystal missing or out of place the next morning (no matter what the fairies and foxes may do at night!).

Intent

Hold your crystal in your hands and imagine a golden light from above coming down and filling the crystal and cleansing it of all negativity.

Sound

All crystals love sound, and you can use a tuning fork, singing bowl, or Tibetan cymbals to cleanse your crystals. Use your choice of sound by playing the sound over and around your crystal. This is a useful technique for large crystals. You might place one crystal inside a singing bowl.

Reiki

If you are attuned to Reiki you can use it to cleanse your crystals. This can be done by placing the crystals in your hands or holding your hands over the crystal and asking the Reiki to flow to cleanse the crystal. This is also a handy technique for any large or awkward crystals.

WISE WOMAN WAYS

Crystal Cave Meditation

Sit or lie comfortably. Close your eyes. Relax your body and slow your breathing. Imagine walking up a woodland path in the spring sunshine. As you walk, the path becomes progressively steeper. As you come to the crest of the hill, you see an opening to your left, leading to a cave in the side of the hill, partially hidden by flowering bushes. Walk into the cave. The air is cool and you see a sparkle where the walls are covered with black opals and red carnelian, giving off a scarlet glow. Walk through the cave of rich red crystals, absorbing their light. You move into another cave. Slowly, the opals and carnelian give way to tangerine quartz glowing a vibrant orange. Walk through the tangerine quartz, absorbing their light. You're moving deeper down into the earth and into another cave. Slowly, the tangerine quartz gives way to citrine and golden tiger's eye, shining with a sunshiny yellow. Walk through the citrine and golden tiger's eye, absorbing their light. The citrine and golden tiger's eye give way to a cave of rose quartz and rainforest jasper. Walk through the crystals, absorbing their light. The crystals give way to a cave of turquoise crystals. Walk through the turquoise, absorbing its light. The turquoise gives way to walls of blue tiger's eye. Walk through the crystal cave, absorbing their light. Farther down and deeper you go. The crystals give way to an amethyst cave. Walk through the amethyst, absorbing its light. Finally, you walk into the innermost cavern, which is completely covered in pure rock crystal. Sit with your baby for a while in harmony with the healing crystals and the quiet stillness of the earth before returning to the outer world.

Charging Crystals

You will need to recharge your crystals immediately after cleaning them. While your crystal already contains its own unique vibrational energies, those energies can sometimes become low or depleted. When you recharge crystals, you're basically giving them the chance to refresh their ability to focus and expand their energy.

Crystal clusters

Crystal cluster chunks, or caves, are known to be self-charging and will charge other crystals lain upon them.

Sound

Put a crystal near a single-note chime and strike the chime gently several times. This has a harmonizing effect on the crystal. If you like to chant, do so in the presence of your crystals. Put your crystal near a bell and gently produce a sound in it. Instead of using a bell you can use a resonant (tuning) fork.

Reiki charging

If you are a Reiki I practitioner, you can charge your crystals with Reiki energy.

Sunlight

The ultraviolet light from the sun containing the full spectrum of light restores a crystal's energy. CAUTION: The sun will fade many crystals, such as amethyst. Direct hot sun beaming through clear quartz may also be a fire hazard.

Moonlight

Crystals can be recharged using the softened solar radiation reflected via the moon. CAUTION: Be aware of rain if placing outside.

WISE WOMAN WAYS

I have to confess to occasionally needing to cleanse and charge my crystals with not a lot of time to spare. As long as your intent is honourable and clear, it's wonderful how quickly the crystals will oblige! The crystals I have the privilege of working with may be used for teaching or healing. I offer a prayer for protection and of intent, asking that the crystals be cleansed of all negative energy and charged with the blessings of the Goddess for the highest good of all. I then smudge the room and the crystals.

Chakra Balancing With Crystals

One of the simplest ways to use crystals during pregnancy is to balance the chakra system using crystals. To realign chakra energies, place one or two crystals of the appropriate colour on each chakra area for a few minutes.

First (root or base) chakra

How it can help: This will balance physical energy, motivation, and practicality and promote a sense of reality. It's a good idea to place a grounding stone like smoky quartz or black tourmaline between the feet to act as an anchor.

Related quartz crystals: Red tourmaline, onyx, red aventurine, red carnelian, red chalcedony, red-brown agate, ruby aura quartz, rutilated quartz, black smoky quartz, grey banded and Botswana agate, rainbow jasper, red and brecciated jasper, and red tiger's eye.

Second (sacral or spleen) chakra

How it can help: The second chakra is very sensitive during pregnancy and working with this area not only influences your energy field but that of your baby. Placing crystals next to your body rather than directly on the chakra may help balance creativity and release blocks in your life that prevent pleasure.

Related quartz crystals: Carnelian, carnelian agate, drusy quartz, fire agate, fire opal, lepidocrosite included in quartz or amethyst, orange phantom quartz, Oregon opal, red jasper, and chryoprase.

WISE WOMAN WAYS

Stick to the gentler and lighter-coloured crystals, remembering their energies will also pass through to the baby.

- **MOONSTONE** represents the Divine Feminine and is the best stone for supporting you through pregnancy, working with the moon and its cycles, balancing energy, easing through pregnancy, and into childbirth.
- **ROSE QUARTZ** is the unconditional love hug of the Universe. Wrapping yourself and baby in its warm, soothing energy provides emotional balance, security, and peace.
- **CITRINE** offers protection during pregnancy.
- **AMETHYST** in conjunction with LAVENDER ESSENTIAL OIL warmed in a defuser may be used during difficult times throughout your pregnancy.
- **CARNELIAN** or **ROSE QUARTZ** help with pregnancy fatigue.

Third (solar plexus) chakra

How it can help: To reduce anxiety, clear thoughts, and improve overall confidence.

Related quartz crystals: Citrine, spirit quartz, lemon chryoprase, opal aura quartz, smokey citrine, sunshine aura quartz, yellow jasper, yellow phantom quartz, yellow tourmaline, sulphur in quartz, golden healer quartz, rutilated quartz, and golden tiger's eye.

Fourth (heart) chakra

How it can help: To promote a sense of calm, create a sense of direction in life, and balance your relationship with others and the world. A pink stone can be added for emotional clearing.

Related quartz crystals: Aventurine, apple aura quartz, chryoprase, dentric agate, green agate, green aventurine, green jasper, heliotrope, leopardskin jasper (jaguar stone), moss agate, olive jasper, peach aventurine, pink agate, pink carnelian, pink chalcedony, pink tourmaline, rainforest jasper, rose aura quartz, smokey rose quartz, strawberry quartz, green tourmaline, and rose quartz.

Fifth (throat) chakra

How it can help: To bring peace, ease communication difficulties, and promote self-expression.

Related quartz crystals: Aqua aura, blue aventurine, blue chalcedony, blue jasper, blue lace agate, blue phantom quartz, blue tiger's eye, blue-green agate, moss agate, tourmaline, water opal (hyalite), watermelon tourmaline, avalonite (drusy blue chalcedony), and blue agate.

Sixth (brow) chakra

How it can help: To promote intuitive skills and memory and increase understanding and self-knowledge.

Related quartz crystals: Amethyst, blue jasper, blue tiger's eye, chrysophal (blue-green opal) smoky quartz, and moss agate.

Seventh (crown) chakra

How it can help: This will integrate and balance all aspects of the self—physical, mental, emotional, and spiritual—and will promote positive thought patterns, inspiration, and imagination.

Related quartz crystals: Amethyst, amethyst spirit quartz, Botswana agate, lavender quartz, lavender amethyst, rock crystal, moonstone, ametrine, and clear quartz.

> **WISE WOMAN WAYS**
> - **MALACHITE, THE "MIDWIFE'S STONE,"** nurtures the baby in your womb and assists in birthing.
> - **LAPIS LAZULI** alleviates pain at the time of birthing, before and after delivery of baby. Keep as a touch stone or wrap it in a soft white cloth and tie it between your breast and stomach.

Crystals For Different Pregnancy States

Pregnancy State	Quartz Crystal
Apprehension, anxiety, worry	Amethyst, aventurine, clear quartz, rose quartz, smoky quartz, black tourmaline, blue lace agate, watermelon tourmaline, carnelian, green aventurine, Herkimer diamond, siberian quartz, jasper, fire agate, smoky quartz, jasper (chakras: brow, heart, solar plexus)
Constipation	Smoky quartz, black tourmaline
Depression	Amethyst, elestial quartz, smoky quartz, rose quartz, carnelian, amethyst, smoky quartz, black tourmaline, rutilated quartz, lithium quartz, ametrine, Botswana

	agate, carnelian, moss agate, tiger's eye, purple tourmaline, Siberian quartz (chakra: solar plexus)
Fatigue	Clear quartz, yellow jasper, black tourmaline, peru opal, amethyst, rose quartz, carenelian, fire agate, ametrine, blue opal, dendritic agate (chakra: base)
Fuzzy thinking	Clear quartz, black tourmaline, amethyst, smoky quartz, opal, moss agate, green tourmaline, red jasper (chakras: brow, crown)
Indecisive, self-doubting	Carnelian, smoky quartz, tiger's eye
Insomnia	Amethyst, smoky quartz, candle quartz, moonstone, chrysoprase, rose quartz (chakra: brow)
Intolerant, critical, irritable	Rose quartz
Low self-esteem	Rose quartz, moss agate, chrysoberyl, citrine, opal, tourmaline (chakras: base, spleen, heart)
Lack of sexual interest	Carnelian, rose quartz (chakra: brow, base)
Panic	Green tourmaline
Backache	Green tourmaline, blue agate
Nausea or sickness	Moonstone, red jasper
Constipation	Smoky quartz, black tourmaline, red jasper, citrine
Piles/hemerrhoids	Bloodstone
Itching	Green aventurine
Headache	Rose quartz, amethyst, blue lace agate, citrine, moonstone

Water retention	Moonstone
Acidity	Rock crystal, green jasper
Leg cramps	Bloodstone
Sinus	Blue lace agate
Varicose veins	Blue lace agate, bloodstone
Birthing and new beginnings	Moss agate

WISE WOMAN WAYS

Massaging with crystals combines the relaxing benefits of massage with the healing energy of crystals. If feeling stressed or headachy, choose smooth, clear quartz crystals such as spheres (I generally use the smooth end of a wand, one for either side of the head), tumble stones, or palm stones. Circle the crystal gently around the temples and over the forehead.

Ways To Use Crystals

In grids

A crystal grid involves using six single-pointed crystals (I would suggest using clear quartz or amethyst). If you are laying down, place one by your left foot with the point going up, one by your elbow, point up, and one by the left of your head, point up. Then place one by the right of your head point going down, one by your elbow, point down, and one by your right foot, point down.

Placement of the Crystals

If you are sitting in a chair, place a crystal by your left foot going up, one just behind the chair on your left going up, one just behind the chair on your right going down, and one by your right foot, going down. You may choose to hold a crystal in your hand.

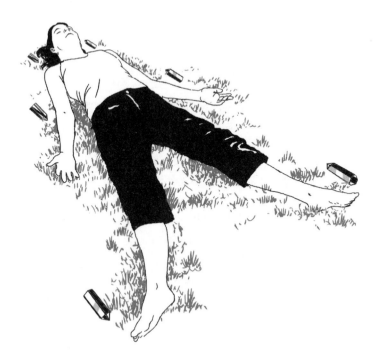

Gem essences

Gem essences can be dropped under the tongue, rubbed into pulse or chakra points, sprayed into the aura, put in bath water, or sprayed around a room. The basic principle behind the use of gem essences is the same as that of flower essences, in that when crystals are activated by natural sunlight or moonlight, they transfer their vibrational signature into water, creating a remedy that is safe and can be used in conjunction with all healing modalities. Once you have your gem essence, you can enhance it with flower essences. Put two drops of the chosen flower essences into the gem mixture. This is a particularly nice way to blend the energies of Bach Flower Remedies or Australian Bush Flower Essences with crystals. **Note:** some crystals are toxic if taken internally.

Other ways to use crystals

You could wear crystals on a waist chain, bracelet or on a chain between your breasts, place it under your pillow, or hold it while meditating. Experiment with placing crystals at strategic points in a room.

> **WISE WOMAN WAYS**
> Make up a crystal power pouch containing the crystals of your choice, plus some sage for cleansing negativity, and carry it with you.

What Happens Next?

Crystals are a gift to you from Mother Earth and can be used as part of your energy healing during pregnancy. Another Wise Woman healing art that uses energy healing is hand reflexology, which you can easily learn and do anywhere to help comfort and sooth any distress of pregnancy. Interested to know more? Then turn the page and read on.

CHAPTER 10

Hand Reflexology
for Pregnancy

Whilst the art of reflexology dates back to Ancient Egypt, India, and China, it wasn't until 1913 that Dr. William Fitzgerald introduced this therapy to the West as Zone Therapy. Dr. Fitzgerald researched how reflex areas on the feet and hands were linked to areas and organs of the body within the same zone. During the 1930s, Eunice Ingham further developed this Zone theory into what is now known as Reflexology, observing that congestion in any part of the foot was mirrored in the corresponding part of the body.

> **WISE WOMAN WAYS**
>
> I treat women with reflexology who:
> - have had miscarriages and want their body to heal in preparation for conception;
> - are going through in vitro fertilization (IVF);
> - are preparing to conceive;
> - have had a normal conception and want reflexology throughout their pregnancy;
> - want to start their birthing naturally.
>
> In addition to classic reflexology, I often show the women how to practice self-treatment using hand reflexology and show the partners how they can use simple foot reflexology on their women.

Reflexology treatments during pregnancy are a natural and gentle way of relieving stress and anxiety and can help prepare your body for childbirth. By enabling a calm, relaxed mind and body, reflexology has been shown to help lessen the chance of being induced and reduce the length of birthing.

What Is Hand Reflexology?

The feet are rich in nerve endings, which are why they are traditionally used by reflexologists to stimulate the flow of energy throughout the body, but the hands (and other key areas of the body) can also be used successfully, as discussed below. Hand reflexology can be self-administered anywhere and can bring ease and comfort during pregnancy.

Caution!

While there are many self-help steps you can take to improve the well-being of yourself and your baby, if you have any concerns about using hand reflexology, consult a qualified reflexologist. I would suggest you use these techniques two weeks before you are due to give birth.

Hand reflexology contraindications

The main hand reflexology contraindications are as follows:
- Don't do it on broken skin on the hands.
- Don't do hand reflexology if you have a hand injury.
- If you have any medical problem, consult a doctor first.
- If you can't use your fingers or knuckles, use the blunt end of a pencil or the blunt end of a crystal wand.

Hand reflexology techniques

You may use all these techniques in one session, or just one technique:

1. RUBBING: Briskly rubbing your palms together will generate energy (chi) in them.

2. SQUEEZING: Using your thumb pad and index finger to firmly squeeze each finger and thumb on the other hand, from base to tip.

3. PULLING: Using your thumb pad and index finger to firmly grasp the base of each finger and thumb on the other hand and pull down towards the tip.

4. PRESSING: Using the tip of your thumb to press and stimulate points on the opposite hand (you will need short nails!). Press until you feel pressure. Hold the pressure and work the point with rotary, or circular, pressure.

4. ROTARY, OR CIRCULAR, PRESSURE: Press into the point and move in very small firm circles using a knuckle of the other hand or the blunt end of a pencil or crystal wand. I would recommend a rose quartz wand with a little essential oil on the blunt end (not too much oil though, or the wand will slip).

5. THUMB ROLL: Rolling the pad of your thumb over the points, massage the relevant points on both hands a couple of times a day.

> **WISE WOMAN WAYS**
> You could put a flower essences mixture in the centre of your palms before giving yourself hand reflexology. Or mix a little essential oil in with some hand cream and rub into your hands before giving yourself hand reflexology. Not too much, otherwise your fingers will skid everywhere!

Self-treatment

1. Begin by sitting quietly and closing your eyes. Take a few deep breaths as you still your body and focus your mind.

2. Begin your hand reflexology treatment by pinching the tips of each finger of your left hand (nail to back). Reverse and repeat on your right hand. A few seconds for each finger tip will do. EXTREME CAUTION: *Avoid both thumbs. There is a point here for the pituitary gland, which releases oxytocin, the hormone that kick-starts birthing. You can massage this point two weeks before due date.*

3. After pinching the tops of your finger tips, go back to each tip and pinch them again, this time squeezing from side to side of the fingertip.

4. Vigorously rub from base to tip of each finger of your left hand, front and back, plus sides. Reverse and repeat this process on your right hand. Tug each finger and thumb firmly.

5. Using your right thumb and forefinger, firmly grasp the webbed area between your thumb and forefinger of your left hand. Keeping a firm hold, tug at the skin gently until the fleshy web snaps away from your grasp. Repeat this process for the areas between all your fingers. Reverse and repeat this process on your right hand.

6. Turn your left hand palm down. Use your right thumb to massage the back of your hand.

7. Massage the knuckles and in between the knuckle area first. Continue thumb massaging each area on the back of the hand. Reverse and repeat this process on your right hand.

8. Cradle your left wrist (palm up) inside your right hand. Use your thumb to massage your inner wrist. Reverse and repeat this process on your right hand.

9. Massage the palm of your left hand with your right thumb, knuckle, or the blunt end of a crystal wand. Massage the fleshier mound areas more deeply. Reverse and repeat this process on your right hand.

10. At the end of the session press your right thumb or the blunt end of a crystal wand deeply in the center of your left palm. Reverse and repeat this process on your right hand. Take a few deep breaths and center yourself.

Helpful Reflexology Points for Menopause

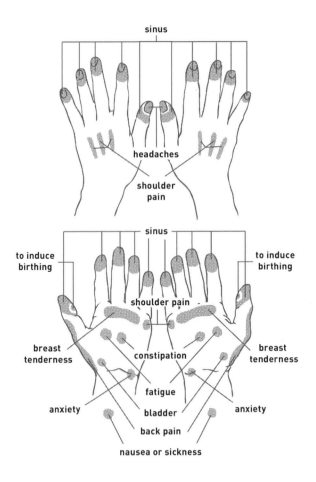

sinus

headaches

shoulder
pain

sinus

to induce
birthing

to induce
birthing

shoulder pain

breast
tenderness

constipation

breast
tenderness

anxiety

fatigue

anxiety

bladder

back pain

nausea or sickness

Specific Pregnancy Points

BACK PAIN: Work the spine points, which run along the outer edge of the thumb down towards the wrist. Apply rotary pressure along this area with the other hand. The point where the centre of your hand joins your wrist can be stimulated to give relief from lower back pain.

BREAST TENDERNESS: Work the breast reflex on the left hand (top of hands under fingers) by rubbing with firm pressure, using the thumb of the right hand. Reverse and repeat this process on your right hand.

SHOULDER PAIN: Part of the shoulder reflex is on both palms of the hand under the little finger, which can be worked with a rotary pressure. Working the reflex points on the backs of the hands in the grooves between the long bones will ease tension over and between the shoulder blades. To work them, use your fingertips. If your left shoulder is the problem, work the reflex points on your left hand. Put your right thumb flat on your left palm. On the back of your left hand, place the tips of your right index, middle, and ring fingers in the grooves. Gently apply and maintain even pressure, slowly and repeatedly moving your fingertips in the direction of the wrist. Reverse and repeat on the right hand.

SINUS: Squeeze and pull around the sinus reflex points on the top third of each finger and thumb (completely around the finger and thumb) on both hands.

BLADDER: With your left palm up, the bladder point is just above where the base of the thumb joins the wrist. Apply pressure to this point with your thumb or knuckle. Reverse and repeat on the right hand.

FATIGUE: Work the adrenal reflex on the left hand with your right. Find the webbing between thumb and index finger and go into the palm about an inch. Apply a rotary pressure on the area indicated, using the thumb or knuckle of the right hand. Reverse and repeat this process on your right hand. Do not work this reflex if you have high blood pressure.

HEADACHES: Apply rotary pressure all around the nail area of the left thumb with your other hand. Reverse and repeat on the right hand

ANXIETY: Find the skin crease that runs right across your wrist at the base of your hand. The point is almost at the medial end of the crease, just inside the edge of the wrist bone (little finger side). Use your thumb pad to press the point until you feel a strong pressure. Hold the pressure while you knead the point using rotary movements for about 1 minute. Repeat on the other wrist. Press both points 2–3 times a day or and whenever you feel anxious.

> **WISE WOMAN WAYS**
>
> If the pregnancy sickness is made worse with movement, listen to a MorningWell CD (www.morningwell.co.uk), which uses specially designed music with underlying frequent pulsations, aimed at reconditioning the balancing mechanism in your inner ear.

NAUSEA OR SICKNESS: I'm using an acupressure tip for this one. With your left palm up, measure three fingers width (using your right hand) down from the first crease where your wrist bends. Where your index finger falls, feel along the crease for a slight dip in the groove between the two large tendons. Apply pressure at that point with your thumb and index finger (both sides of the wrist) for one to two minutes. Repeat with your other hand.

CONSTIPATION: Massage the dip in the palms of both hands with a clockwise movement.

TO INDUCE BIRTHING: Stimulating the point for the pituitary gland will release the hormone oxytocin, which kick-starts birthing. Find the pituitary gland reflex on the center of the thumbprint swirl on the left hand and apply rotary pressure on this point. Reverse and repeat this process on your right hand. EXTREME CAUTION: *Do not use until one week before your due date.*

Note: The ears (like the feet and hands) contain reflexology points corresponding to major body parts and areas. To work with these points, sit with your back straight and use your thumbs and your index fingers to rub and gently pull your ears from the top to bottom. You can also use the tips of your index fingers to rub the inside surface of both ears. Start at the ear opening and work your way to the outside edge, rubbing all the curves and folds of each ear, including behind your ears. Do this for 1–2 minutes per ear.

WISE WOMAN WAYS

Sometimes my lower back gets a little temperamental, so I use hand reflexology to ease the discomfort. I tend to use my knuckles (especially the corner of a knuckle), and I use very small movements as I move down the spinal area on the thumbs.

What Happens Next?

Let's move from the body-centred focus of the last few chapters to a place where you can create rituals to celebrate and honour your pregnancy journey.

CHAPTER 11

Creating Rituals

Rituals provide us with a sense of security and stability—from planting the spring bulbs to celebrating Yuletide. Ritual is different to habit. Habit, such as walking the dog, can be mindless but necessary, while ritual is an intentional, focused action. Ritual can create significance and celebration throughout pregnancy and offers opportunities to create harmony, patience, and appreciation in our lives.

Creating Sacred Space

Space is all around us. It can be full or empty. It can be literal (the kitchen) or abstract (our mind). Sacred can mean a special place to commune with yourself and the Divine, whether it be God, Goddess, or something else. It is a space to be treated with reverence, set apart from the mundane. We can create a sacred space anywhere we choose—inside a building or outside in nature.

WISE WOMAN WAYS

Stand naked in front of a mirror by candlelight and create your anointing oil by mixing pure olive oil with frankincense or sandalwood. Ground and protect yourself and cast your sacred space. Take a drop of your mixture on your index finger and touch each chakra in turn while saying the following aloud:

- **CROWN:** Bless me, Mother Goddess, that my spirit may be clear and true.

- **THIRD EYE:** Bless my inner vision, that I may see with insight.
- **THROAT:** Bless my self-expression, that I may speak with wisdom.
- **HEART:** Bless my heart, that it be open and filled with compassion.
- **SOLAR PLEXUS:** Bless my sense of self-esteem, that I may be true to myself.
- **SACRAL:** Bless my womb, that I may connect with my baby.
- **ROOT:** Bless my yoni, the gateway of life and death.
- **BOTTOMS OF FEET:** Bless my feet, that I may symbolically walk the path of motherhood with courage.
- **PALMS OF HANDS:** Bless my hands, that I may symbolically give with unconditional love.

Casting your circle of sacred space

What we are doing when we cast a circle of sacred space is defining an area to be used for contemplation, meditation, or healing. This is the method I use when I am creating a sacred space. You can adapt it to suit your own needs:

1. Cleanse your area of work by, for example, smudging the area, use your besom (broom) to symbolically clear away negativity, or using "singing bowls" to clear the space.
2. Ground and protect yourself.
3. Have everything inside your circle that you are likely to need.
4. Stand facing outwards at the eastern point. Place your hands together at the heart chakra, and bring your hands up to a point above your head as far as you can go. Say (silently or otherwise):

"Guardian of the East and the element of Air, I call upon your presence and protection during this sacred healing." As you say the words, draw your hands apart in a wide circle until they meet palms and fingertips together at your second (sacral) chakra. Walk to the southern point.

5. Stand facing outwards at the southern point. Place your hands together at the heart chakra, and bring your hands up to a point above your head as far as you can go. Say (silently or otherwise): "Guardian of the South and the element of Fire, I call upon your presence and protection during this sacred healing." As you say the words, draw your hands apart in a wide circle until they meet palms and fingertips together at your second (sacral) chakra. Walk to the western point.

6. Stand facing outwards at the western point. Place your hands together at the heart chakra, and bring your hands up to a point above your head as far as you can go. Say (silently or otherwise): "Guardian of the West and the element of Water, I call upon your presence and protection during this sacred healing." As you say the words, draw your hands apart in a wide circle until they meet palms and fingertips together at your second (sacral) chakra. Walk to the northern point.

7. Stand facing outwards at the northern point. Place your hands together at the heart chakra, and bring your hands up to a point above your head as far as you can go. Say: "Guardian of the North and the element of Earth, Lord and Lady/God and Goddess, I call upon your presence and protection during this sacred healing." As you say the words, draw your hands apart in a wide circle until they meet palms and fingertips together at your second (sacral) chakra. Walk to the eastern point.

8. Stand facing inwards at the eastern point, and point from where you are with the index finger of your dominant hand or with a

crystal wand. Trace a clockwise circle of protection around you (and the other person if appropriate) or altar. Visualize the circle strong and protective around you, going deep down into the Earth and upwards to the sky. Ask the God and Goddess (of your choice) that all within the circle come under the full protection of the God and Goddess at all times.

9. When the circle is complete with your energy, you should declare what the circle is for. A statement that this circle is created in love and compassion for self-healing for example.

> **WISE WOMAN WAYS**
>
> I find a certain amount of comfort in ritual. Maybe, it's the familiarity and safety that allow creative energy to build. However, it's also true that stepping into the energetic abyss armed with good grounding and protection can invite a level of inspiration unavailable when dealing with the purely familiar.

Having cast your circle, you must always close it after your work is complete. This is the method I use. Again, you can adapt it to suit own your own needs:

1. Stand facing outwards at the eastern point. Place your hands together at the heart chakra, and bring your hands up to a point above your head as far as you can go. Say (silently or otherwise): "Guardian of the East and the element of Air, I thank you for your presence and protection during this sacred healing. I bid you farewell." As you say the words, draw your hands apart in a wide circle until they meet palms and fingertips together at your second (sacral) chakra. Walk to the southern point.

2. Stand facing outwards at the southern point. Place your hands together at the heart chakra, and bring your hands up to a point above your head as far as you can go. Say (silently or otherwise): "Guardian of the South and the element of Fire, I thank you for your presence and protection during this sacred healing. I bid you farewell." As you say the words, draw your hands apart in a wide circle until they meet palms and fingertips together at your second (sacral) chakra. Walk to the western point.

3. Stand facing outwards at the western point. Place your hands together at the heart chakra, and bring your hands up to a point above your head as far as you can go. Say (silently or otherwise): "Guardian of the West and the element of Water, I thank you for your presence and protection during this sacred healing. I bid you farewell." As you say the words, draw your hands apart in a wide circle until they meet palms and fingertips together at your second (sacral) chakra. Walk to the northern point.

4. Stand facing outwards at the northern point. Place your hands together at the fourth (heart) chakra, and bring your hands up to a point above your head as far as you can go. Say (silently or otherwise): "Guardian of the North and the element of Earth, God, and Goddess (or your choice), I thank you for your presence and protection during this sacred healing. I bid you farewell." As you say the words, draw your hands apart in a wide circle until they meet palms and fingertips together at your second (sacral) chakra. Walk to the eastern point.

5. Stand facing inwards at the eastern point, and point from where you are with your dominant hand, palm down and fingers outstretched, or use a crystal wand. Trace an anti-clockwise circle around you and the other person or altar. Visualize the circle melting around you.

Although I have done many rituals in a modest way, I was nervous about casting my first circle. In fact, it was only after I had a dream where I was casting a circle that I began doing it for real. Even now, I am private in my rituals. A couple of years ago, I was doing a ritual alone in the garden, arms outstretched upwards—going great guns. I heard a noise behind me and saw my husband who had come home early from work, sitting quietly watching me. Although I know Mick has great respect for my beliefs, I still found it difficult when I knew he was watching.

WISE WOMAN WAYS

A birth altar helps set your focus for pregnancy rituals, ceremonies, and healing. This space should be large enough for you to conduct your work upon. It might be a permanent table or a table you put up and take down for use anywhere. I have "spaces" rather than altars. For example, there are spaces in my healing room for crystals. On the nightstand next to my side of the bed is an amethyst crystal with some night-time Rescue Remedy, plus a homeopathic remedy (all energy medicine). When the mood takes me, I put some flowers and greenery from the garden there as well, so the last thing I see at night is nature (or my lovely husband or maybe one of my four black cats peering down at me!). You may choose to represent the four elements on your birth altar or sacred space with the following suggested articles:

- **AIR:** candles, feathers, smudge stick
- **FIRE:** candle, incense, a small cauldron, smudge stick, an oil burner, a vessel to burn herbs
- **WATER:** floating candle, flowers in water, a ritual chalice with water

> • **EARTH:** plant, a small branch, crystals/gems, a vessel to burn herbs
>
> Consider adding eggs, seeds, or a growing plant to symbolize the new life carried within you.
>
> Before you begin any ritual, you should cleanse the area where the work is to be done and then cast the circle, as noted above. Once your work is complete, shut down the energy used for your workings, as discussed earlier, by thanking the guides, teachers, or God/Goddess that you called or who came into the circle to offer assistance. Then imagine the energy around the circle lowering around you fading. Finally, clear the space with a blessing and ask the energies to close the spiritual gateways.

Daily Rituals And Pregnancy

As we journey through pregnancy, we need to have time for ourselves, time for bonding with baby, and maybe time for being with our partner as a family unit. Some ways in which we may do this:

- Prepare good food and eat mindfully.
- Engage in daily nature breaks.
- Restore rest periods during the day.
- Let go of things that take up space, require maintenance, and make decision-making more complicated.
- Let go of important tasks that someone else can do.
- Indulge in regular child's play. Indulge in a craft project. Sit quietly and daydream.
- Begin your weekly planning by considering the activities you choose to care for your physical, spiritual, mental, and social well-being.

- Walk, exercise, or do some pregnancy yoga. Enjoy a massage; take a sauna; get your hair done; have a facial, pedicure, or manicure; take a warm bath by candlelight before snuggling down in bed.
- Be with your partner and share what brings you both joy and pleasure as two adults.
- Share your motherhood with your partner and celebrate their role in parenthood.

Ritual For Creating A Pregnancy Ceremony

Do you want to create a ceremony for pregnancy? Why do you want to mark it? If you would like to enable healing, what healing and why? If you wish to strengthen and solidify a relationship, what kind of relationship and how do you want to strengthen or solidify it? Maybe you wish to create a ceremony to welcome the spirit of the baby or to celebrate the bonding of parent to baby. It could be that you would like to state your beliefs and express your hope for the future. What beliefs? What are your hopes?

Preparing for the ceremony

Where would you like the ceremony? Who would you like to witness the ceremony? Do you want any special clothing?

Opening the ceremony

You might like to include candle lighting, music, essential oils or incense, a blessing, or a statement of intent.

Main body of the ceremony

You might like to include candle lighting, blessing of liquid/food, chanting, drumming, meditation, essential oils or incense, hand or foot washing, planting something, making a gift of charity, making a vow of service, reading text, storytelling, exchanging or giving gifts, creating amulets, singing, music, dancing, prayers and blessings, immersion in water, anointing, guided meditation or visualization, silence, and the use of ritual objects.

Closing the ceremony

You could close with a blessing, music, or sharing of food and drink.

WISE WOMAN WAYS

Have a Blessing Way on the full moon before your due date. Lighting a candle at the Blessing Way is a lovely way to bring a sacred feel to the atmosphere or you can ask each guest to bring a candle to light during their blessing for you. Afterwards each guest will take her candle home and light it when she hears you are birthing. During this ritual, your friends and family brush your hair and bathe your feet with herbs, such as sage for wisdom, bay for protection, and calendula for sacred affection. Each woman in the circle comes forward to present you with a prayer, poem, or blessing. Another idea is to ask each guest to bring a bead they have picked for you. At the blessing all the beads are strung onto a cord for you to wear during birthing. A belly cast is a fun activity that can be done at the Blessing Way. It also gives you a lovely keepsake of your body full of baby. Finish the Blessing Way with shared food and drink.

What Happens Next?

The energies of you and your baby are melded. Your mind, body, and spirit are ripe for birthing. Let's move into wise woman birthing.

JANE'S JOURNEY

I used ritual at least twice during my work with Laurel. The first time was when I was going through my second cycle and was becoming overwhelmed with the self-administration of some of the drugs. Laurel suggested creating a loving, comfortable ritual in order to administer a key injection to myself. Entering into this gentle, female space helped me to honour the (medical) journey I was taking. Another time was just at the end of the first trimester, when we talked about me allowing daily nourishing time with baby.

CHAPTER 12

Wise Woman Birthing

This is your birthing time. You have choices about how you experience the joy of bringing your child into the world.

Caution!

While there are many self-help steps you can take to improve the well-being of yourself and your baby, if you have any concerns about homeopathy, aromatherapy, or herbs, consult a qualified practitioner. Here are some wise woman ways you might like to use during your birthing.

> **WISE WOMAN WAYS**
> When you go into birthing, light a candle to illuminate your path. Ask those who care for you to light candles for you and your baby, as well.

Homeopathy

Homeopathy can help during all stages of the birthing process as well as in the after-birth. A wonderful kit called The Essential 7 Little Birth Kit is available from The Little Birth Kit Company *(www.littlebirthkits.com)*. The kit includes full instructions on how and when to use the remedies.

Herbs

(use only under the guidance of a qualified herbalist)

ANGELICA ROOT is a powerful uterine stimulant and can help expel the placenta.

BLUE AND BLACK COHOSH can be used for induction.

COMFREY is a herb that can be used externally to encourage healing and prevent infection if you have a perineal tear.

EVENING PRIMROSE OIL helps to soften the cervix by providing prostaglandins that encourage birthing and the components the body needs to make prostaglandins. Evening primrose oil can be used internally near the end of pregnancy by being massaged directly onto the cervix (squeeze oil out of capsule onto a clean finger and massage the cervix). **Note:** Evening primrose oil should not be taken orally until after 37 weeks of pregnancy.

RASPBERRY LEAF: Drinking this as a tea or taking as a tincture during birthing may help stimulate stronger surges. Drink after the birthing to stimulate milk production and assist your uterus in returning to pre-pregnancy size.

WISE WOMAN WAYS

Wear a jasper pendant on a black cord between your breasts to help your milk come through.

Preparing The Environment

By creating a quiet, safe, and intimate setting, you will have the space to get in touch with your wise woman wisdom so that you and your baby can have a positive birth experience. Whether you plan to give birth at home, in a birth centre, or in a hospital, create an environment that is as sacred and nurturing as possible.

PRIVACY: Consider the availability of privacy at your birthing place. How comfortable might you feel making noise?

WATER: Water can be a comfort during birthing. How easy will it be for you to access a bath or shower?

SOUNDS: Does your birthing place have a way for you to play CDs?

LIGHTING: Most women prefer a dimly lit or dark room when

birthing. Can the lighting in your birthing place be adapted or adjusted? Can you use candles?

FRESH AIR: Does your birthing place have a garden in which you can walk, or windows that can be opened? You may want to bring a fan.

WISE WOMAN WAYS

You might want to use the following massage blends, which can be made up by diluting five drops of essential oil in 5mls of base oil:

- **FRANKINCENSE** to alleviate fear;
- **ROSEMARY** to push past fatigue;
- **PEPPERMINT** to alleviate nausea during transition;
- **JUNIPER BERRY** to stimulate the uterus if surges are dwindling (particularly in second stage);
- **JASMINE** to ease birth pains and dispel placenta.

Birthing Partners

A birthing partner can be a wonderful support during the hours before your baby is in your arms. They can entertain you, hold you, encourage you, massage you, feed you, cool your brow, make you laugh, provide emotional support, or be a shoulder to chew on (I've seen this happen!). The birthing partner can intercede in medical interventions where appropriate. They can reassure you, comfort you, become your eyes and ears, and remind you of what to do and how well you are doing it. A birthing partner could be your friend, your mother, your partner, your sister, or anyone you trust.

You might choose to have a doula (a Greek word meaning "women's servant") with you during your birth. Some doulas have clinical skills while others are trained in hypnobirthing. Your doula can either perform comfort measures for you or help your birthing partners to support you.

WISE WOMAN WAYS
During the month before birthing, ritualize your days around the goddesses of birth (see page 21).

Mindset And Birthing

Using positive images will deepen the mind-body link during birthing. The more powerfully you can visualize a positive image in your mind, the stronger the connection to your body and baby.

Some ideas:

- Visualize your baby smoothly moving down to come into your arms.
- Centre on a comforting image during surges, such as a sanctuary where you are birthing your baby with ease and comfort.
- Visualize your cervix opening like a rose for your baby to come through.
- Imagine the waves rolling and breaking on the beach and then pausing before moving again.
- Imagine you and your baby are immersed in warm, blue water that is gently rocking you both into a safe harbour.

WISE WOMAN WAYS
Look for "opening" symbols that mean birthing to you: a labyrinth, the full moon, a budding flower, a bowl, a lotus, or a circle. Use the symbol as a focal point during the birth.

Using positive thinking

Just as you might pack essential oils or soothing music into your birth pack, choose to pack your mind with positive statements like:

- I am happy that my baby is finally coming to me.
- I am focused on a smooth and easy birth.
- I trust my body to know what it needs to do.
- My mind and body are relaxed.
- I feel confident. I feel safe. I feel secure.
- The baby is moving down. The baby will be here soon.
- My body is working perfectly. Everything is working perfectly.
- My muscles work in complete harmony to make birthing easier.
- My baby moves gently along in its journey.
- Each surge of my body brings my baby closer to me.
- I meet each surge with my breath. My body is at ease.
- I release my birthing over to my body and my baby.

> **WISE WOMAN WAYS**
> Create your own birthing mantra of two or three sentences. Use it at different times during the birthing to meet your baby. While chanting the mantra, visualize a circle slowly pulsing larger.

Natural Pain Management

Try the following natural pain management techniques:

Frozen water bottle

Fill a flat-sided, plastic water bottle with water and freeze (you could always pop some Bach Flower Rescue Remedy in the water before freezing). Lean against something and place the bottle at your lower back to ease pain. Keep several water bottles in the freezer. As the ice melts, take sips of the cold water and replace the bottle with another frozen water bottle.

Baths and showers

In the shower, the warmth and pressure of the water aimed at your lower back will help relieve tension in the muscles. Kneel in the shower and rest your upper body on a birth ball. In a bath, you will find the water helps to support the weight of the uterus. Keep the water at body temperature.

Tennis balls

Tennis balls help distribute pressure evenly during a counter-pressure massage. Place two tennis balls in a sock. Lean back on a wall and place the tennis balls at your lower back so they provide pressure as you lean on the wall. You can move to roll the balls for more or less pressure.

A rolling pin

Roll the rolling pin up and down your lower back, leaning on the rolling pin to add more pressure.

> **WISE WOMAN WAYS**
>
> Australian Bush Flower Essences for birthing include:
>
> - **CROWEA, BOTTLEBRUSH,** and **BAUHINIA,** taken together, may help you move from the first to second stage of birthing. Bottlebrush will also help you bond with your baby.
> - **ESSENCE OF BOAB,** given to your baby, will help ease the possibility of difficult emotional patterns being passed on.
> - **SUNDEW** brings your baby's spirit into his or her body.
> - **KAPOK BUSH** and **MACROCARPA** may be used for stamina during the birth.
> - **SLENDER RICE FLOWER** helps you heal from a caesarian section.

Wheat bag

The warmth of a wheat bag can help to minimize the pain of tense muscles during birthing. A wheat bag can also be used as a cold pack by placing the bag in the freezer for a few hours. Stretch the wheat bag under your belly for relief of cervical discomfort. You could drape the bag on your shoulders to help remove neck tension. You could have two wheat bags—one in the freezer and one ready for the microwave!

Breathing

Centre on the breath, breathing deeply and slowly during a surge. Take the advice of your doula or midwife for the pushing and crowning stage. A relaxed mouth and jaw means a relaxed vagina! Personally speaking, when I have a routine cervical smear, I tend to clench so tightly a peanut couldn't pass through! I found that relaxing the bum relaxes the cervix and vagina area as well. Easier to say than do at the time, I appreciate!

> **WISE WOMAN WAYS**
> **MOVING BABY INTO A BETTER POSITION –** The lunge technique encourages the baby to move into a better position as it widens one side of the pelvis and puts pressure on the other. During a surge, place one foot on a chair, couch, or stool, with your knee pointing out. Slowly bend at the hip towards the raised knee, holding the stretch for 10 seconds, then rest for 10 seconds. Continue the lunge-rest-lunge sequence until the surge is over. After a couple of surges, lunge with your other leg.

A birth ball

Ball sitting is comfortable as it allows rest for your legs while still requiring movement in the pelvis. The movement helps baby to find the best position to travel down and into the birth canal. If you feel able during surges, rock the ball gently to help the baby move down the pelvis. Or, when sitting on the ball, and with your birthing partner supporting your upper body, sway your hips from side to side.

Rebozo

The rebozo is a traditional Mexican shawl long enough to wrap around a body with length over (or you could use a large scarf). When used by a birthing partner, the rebozo acts like an extension of their arms allowing them to support your weight.

- POSITION ONE: Sit in an upright position and place the rebozo under your arms and over your chest. The birthing partner stands behind you, holding the ends of the rebozo to support your weight as they gently sway you.
- POSITION TWO: Get in a hands-and-knees position. Wrap the rebozo under your belly and around your thighs, so that your birthing partner can hold the ends above you and gently sway the rebozo side to side.

> **WISE WOMAN WAYS**
> **NIPPLE STIMULATION FOR SLOW BIRTHING –** Oxytocin, the birthing hormone that causes surges, is released in the body when the breasts are stimulated. To stimulate the release of oxytocin, you need to mimic the suckling of a baby through massaging the areola (dark circle around the nipple). Rub the areola in a gentle rolling way with your palm or fingers between surges. Massage one breast at a time, for five minutes and wait 10 minutes to see the effect before continuing. TIP: You could also do this stimulation to induce birthing.

Positions

The position you choose for birthing can affect your comfort and how quickly your body is able to progress in birthing.

Upright positions

Stay upright and active during your birthing as much as possible to decrease birthing time and increase the efficiency of the cervix opening. Upright positions include:

- SQUATTING: Squatting realigns the pelvis to increase the opening at the bottom and uses the force of gravity to help baby move down the birth canal. As a surge begins, move into a squatting position. Bend at the hips and knees until your bottom is close to the floor. Keep your heels on the floor. If you are resting on a bed, bring your knees back and place the soles of your feet on the bed, then move forward into a squat for the pushing surge. At the end of the surge, resume the most comfortable position.

> **WISE WOMAN WAYS**
>
> Buy or make a stuffed toy that you find inspirational and/or comforting. Soak a cotton ball in an essential oil, such as lavender, and sew it into the toy. Infuse the toy with healing energies and thoughts for a calm and safe birthing. You can use the stuffed toy as a focus during birthing and know that your protection and healing energy is with you.

- DANGLING: The dangle position is an upright supported squat that allows your birthing partner to support you. Your birthing partner can sit on a kitchen worktop or bed, with their feet supported on chairs. With your back to the birthing partner, position yourself between their legs. Put your arms over the birthing partner's thighs, and lower yourself into a squatting position, allowing your arms and the birthing partner's legs to support your weight.

- LEANING: The leaning position takes pressure off your pelvic floor and allows the baby to change position. Try leaning while you stand or kneel over a chair, over a birth ball, into someone's lap, over the side of the bath, or over the side or end of a bed.

- MOVING THE PELVIS: Positions that give you the freedom to move your pelvis may help your baby to rotate, allowing for a faster birth, for example:
  - Slow dancing with a partner for support;
  - Swaying your hips back and forth during surges;
  - Rocking your hips in a figure eight during surges (belly dancing is a fab preparation for this one);
  - Pelvic rocking in any of the upright or leaning positions;
  - Rocking your torso back and forth as you sit;
  - Lunging forward with your foot on a chair or stool;
  - Walking in between or during surges.

WISE WOMAN WAYS

Get in the rhythm of using your breath to manage pain by:

- Firstly, establishing a deep and steady breathing rhythm from the abdomen;
- Secondly, breathing out resistance and breathing in peace (thank you, Jane);
- Thirdly, focusing your awareness on the point of pain and breathing through this point in as relaxed a manner as possible to dissolve the hurt.

Sitting positions

These positions allow your body to work with gravity while allowing you to rest. You can sit on a chair facing forward or backward. You could sit on the floor or on a birth ball.

Reclining

These positions allow you to rest between surges. You can recline in bed or on a couch or with pillows on the floor. You can also recline onto a partner who is sitting behind you. If you want to birth in water, you can use the recliner sitting position by using rolled towels or bath pillows.

Side lying

These positions allow you to rest between surges. Using pillows, you can lay on your side on a couch, a bed, or the floor. Side lying supports the weight of the uterus, and allows it to come forward during surges easily. If you prefer to be in water, you can relax on your side using a towel or bath pillow to support your head on the side of the pool or bath.

Hands and knees

The hands-and-knees position helps to relieve pressure on the back. Birthing on hands and knees and doing pelvic rocking can move baby into the pelvis. Alternatively, kneel over a birthing ball with your upper body on the ball, moving your body to keep your balance.

Knee-to-chest

The knee-to-chest position is a variation of the hands-and-knees position, in which your bottom is higher than your shoulders. Begin by getting into a hands-and-knees position. Lower your shoulders to the floor, resting your head sideways on a cushion or pillow. Move your knees farther apart, causing your bottom to lower slightly. Keeping your bottom higher than your shoulders will widen the pelvis. While in the knee-to-chest position, your birthing partner could massage your lower back. You could place a rebozo under your belly before you move into the knee-to-chest position. Once you are in position, your birthing partner can pull up on both ends of the rebozo to relieve some of the weight.

Tug-of-war

The tug-of-war position encourages you to push effectively. You and your birthing partner could pull on a rebozo or towel. By pulling against a force, you use the abdominal muscles necessary for proper pushing. Get into a semi-reclining or squatting position. Hold one end of a towel or rebozo while your birthing partner holds the other. During a surge, you and your birthing partner pull on your respective ends of the towel at the same time. Be sure you are properly supported, so you will not lose your balance.

> **WISE WOMAN WAYS**
> **THE BIRTHING DANCE** - The birth dance (with or without music) is an upright position that encourages baby to move deeper into the pelvis. You and your birthing partner face each other. Put your arms around your birthing partner's shoulders and neck, resting your head where you can depending on height. Your birthing partner's arms will go around your abdomen, clasping hands around your back. Once in position, you and your birthing partner sway together. While birth dancing, your birthing partner can provide a pressure massage on your lower back. Getting into deep breathing will encourage deeper relaxation.

WISE WOMAN WAYS

PLANTING YOUR PLACENTA - In the West, the human placenta tends to be seen as human waste, but in many cultures the placenta is revered for its symbolism of life and spirit and is often buried outside.

For example, the Mossi culture (African) bury the placenta under a tree— Zan boku means "the place where the placenta is buried." The New Zealand Maori plant the placenta with a tree on family land as a gift to Papa Tua Nuku (Mother Earth). In Maori, the word for land and placenta are the same: whenua. Traditional Navajo in the US Southwest also plant the placenta (with a peach tree over it), to remind the family of their particular home place.

If you are burying a fresh placenta under a tree, you might want to wait a few months before planting (keep frozen—but don't confuse it with your lamb chops at suppertime), as the nutrients and hormones within the placenta are so concentrated, they may kill the tree. November–February is the best time to plant, if you are in the UK. Mark the centre of the planting hole and draw out a circle from the centre 1m (3.3ft) in diameter. Dig around the perimeter of the circle and remove the turf to a depth of 5cm (2in). Remove the soil from the hole to the depth of the rootball of the tree. Fork over the base of the hole to break up any compacted areas of soil. Put the placenta in and cover with about 2.5cm (1in) of soil before returning the tree to the hole. Place a piece of wood across the centre of the hole, which should meet the base of the trunk where the trunk and compost join to ensure the tree is planted at the right depth. Tease out a few roots to stop them circling the rootball. Add a handful of fertilizer to the planting hole. Mix some compost with the soil previously removed from the hole and spread this around the rootball. Tread the soil firmly up to the previous planting level. Once filled, water in well. As the placenta breaks down in the soil, the tree will reap the benefits of all the nutrients packed in the placenta. (Thanks to *www. gardenersworld.com* for the advice on how to plant a small tree.)

What Next?

Sweet lady, we've walked together through this book, you, your baby, and me. I wish you and your child all the blessings under the heavens. May you and yours walk in peace until the end of time.

Useful Resources

Organizations

Doula UK, *http://doula.org.uk.*
Doula US, *www.dona.org*

Bex's Story

My intentions for birthing my baby were for it to be as it is—natural. I asked Clare, my friend, and Laurel, who I had visited for Reiki and reflexology, to be my birthing partners. I wanted the sacredness of birthing to be held, and I felt they were the right partners to have.

Laurel's first suggestion was for us to make a birth plan. Planning is not my strong point, and it felt better to change the word "plan" to "intentions." It was necessary to draw up my birthing intentions so that my birthing partners and midwives were clear on how I intended to go about birthing. It also enabled me to prepare and organize for the birth.

I had a birthing pool up in my bedroom for weeks, greeting me each morning with a reminder that things were about to change. I stocked up on energy foods, homeopathic remedies (to be dished out by Laurel), and essential oils—all to assist in a gentle and calm birth. Occasionally, I had reflexology and Reiki treatments from Laurel to deepen the bond between myself and baby. After the "due date" I had reflexology more frequently, to remind baby that sometime soon is probably best!

I felt my first twinges early morning, and I felt glad, excited, and, considering my life situation (which was not easy at the time), calm and ready for this precious journey. I slept a little longer and spent much of the sunny, warm day under the shade of a tree in the local park. Clare and Laurel joined me—which was ideal for getting into a rhythm with each other. Having the space to walk around, stretch, and crouch was a blessing.

By mid-afternoon, I felt things speeding up and change within myself. I needed to be at home—although the outdoors appealed for birthing, maybe it's not ideal! Laurel picked up on baby's energy saying it felt like fine silver rain coming through my own more solid energy field. At home, Clare and Laurel filled the birthing pool—I didn't feel I wanted to use it at that point, but they wisely filled it should I change my mind (I didn't). My surges were by now strong, and I was feeling quiet and inward—listening to my body and baby. I was sometimes visualizing my birth canal as hands which gently guided my baby safely down.

By now, I felt like I had three birthing partners: Clare, keeping me cool with a wet flannel and reminding me I was having a baby and not being off my head on (magic) mushrooms; Laurel, massaging my lower back and handing out homeopathic remedies; and the birthing ball, taking the weight and allowing me to move my pelvis effortlessly.

After the birthing ball, I discovered an even nicer support—Laurel! I think it was meant to be a hug, but I didn't let go! I was breathing down with the surges, and with each one, we both sank down from the knees leaning into each other. It was instinctual, and I found it greatly reassuring, as I felt strong and safe, which enabled me to really connect with my body and baby.

After that it gets harder to put into words, because I was at the mercy of my body and there was nothing going on for me other than surges and the spaces between surges. Once I transitioned the midwife was called, and she arrived whilst I was pushing—though I would describe it as a downward surge in my body, which had its own life force and which I aided by breathing in rhythm.

I was on the bed (fortunately, this was a mattress on the floor) on my hands and knees, squatting, declaring I was HOT—and yeah, I was cursing! Unfortunately, I felt the arrival of the midwife to be an intrusion, as she was shouting her predicted arrival time at me (five minutes to go) and everything had become bright (she needed the lights on) and noisy. I was feeling less connected and starting to question if what was happening was right. I hit the wall in my frustration. (The neighbours did bring me flowers later, though!)

When my waters broke there was meconium, which meant the baby may be distressed and in danger of getting blocked airways, so the midwife insisted it was time to get the baby out. I found this difficult to deal with, because that surely was what I was doing. I didn't understand what else she wanted me to do! Looking back, she was probably trying to encourage me, though I didn't appreciate her approach at the time.

The feel of baby's head had me wondering if it was humanly possible to get it out. Then along came another surge and with it sheer determination and surrender to birthing, and eventually—a baby! For me a boy, Phoenix!

A Little Extra From Laurel

To be asked by Bex to be a birthing partner was an honour. I had worked with Clare in the past, so we were familiar with each other, which helped. Sitting in the park by a lovely old tree with Bex and Clare in the sunshine was a wonderful way to bond together before the hard work began. Bex's surges began to gather momentum during the afternoon, and it was thought best to get her back home. I walked back with Bex, and the energy of the baby coming through her auric field was wonderful.

Back home, Clare and I filled the birthing pool with gallons of water to the right temperature. Clare went out and bought half the local corner shop in terms of quick energy foods for all of us. There were homeopathic remedies, glucose tablets, Bach Flower Rescue Remedy in water, and aromatherapy oils in readiness.

Key moments I remember include: massaging Bex's lower back as she leant over the couch, telling her to keep breathing; holding her up, as she dangled in my arms; rubbing her body, as she yelled into the back of the couch; encouraging her to listen to her body; and breathing with her.

When the midwife came, the energy shifted somewhat briskly. At one point, there were two midwives, plus paramedics who were called in response to the meconium issue. However, Bex still had Clare and me by her side. She had no pain relief, and the birth was completely natural, although the conventional healthcare team was an important part of Phoenix's birth.

The moment when Phoenix was born was absolutely amazing and totally sacred in its uniqueness. Bex held Phoenix, and during the following moments while she was birthing the placenta and just following that, she asked me to hold Phoenix. To hold such a newborn was moving beyond words and is a memory I will always treasure. Something of Bex and Phoenix will always be in my energy field, and I thank them both for allowing that to be so.